The Product of Medicine

The Product of Medicine

HOW EFFICIENCY MADE
AMERICAN HEALTH CARE

Caitjan Gainty

Duke University Press   *Durham and London*   2025

© 2025 DUKE UNIVERSITY PRESS. All rights reserved

Typeset in Portrait and Helvetica Neue by Westchester Publishing Services

Library of Congress Cataloging-in-Publication Data
Names: Gainty, Caitjan, [date] author.
Title: The product of medicine : how efficiency made American health care / Caitjan Gainty.
Description: Durham : Duke University Press, 2025. | Includes bibliographical references and index.
Identifiers: LCCN 2024025091 (print)
LCCN 2024025092 (ebook)
ISBN 9781478031604 (paperback)
ISBN 9781478028420 (hardcover)
ISBN 9781478060611 (ebook)
Subjects: LCSH: Medical care—United States—History—20th century. | Medical policy—United States—History—20th century. | Medical care, Cost of—United States. | Medical economics—United States—History—20th century. | Industrial efficiency—Social aspects—United States.
Classification: LCC R152 .G35 2025 (print) | LCC R152 (ebook) |
DDC 338.4/73621—dc23/eng/20250130
LC record available at https://lccn.loc.gov/2024025091
LC ebook record available at https://lccn.loc.gov/2024025092

Cover art: Historical photographs from the Frank and Lillian Gilbreth Collection, Archives Center, National Museum of American History, Smithsonian Institution.

publication supported by a grant from

The Community Foundation for Greater New Haven

as part of the Urban Haven Project

For Lucas

Contents

Acknowledgments xi

Introduction 1

1 The Product 17

2 The Factory 39

3 The Standard 63

4 The Labor 91

5 The Market 115

6 Monopoly 139

Afterword 163

Notes 169
Bibliography 199
Index 221

Acknowledgments

The surgeon and efficiency zealot Ernest Amory Codman opened his treatment on the anatomy of the shoulder with a long, provocative, and wildly entertaining preface. An autobiography-cum-hagiography, it details the peaks and valleys of a life lived slightly outrageously and certainly melodramatically. "If an author has labored to present his material in clear English, properly punctuated and painstakingly illustrated for the benefit of the reader," he wrote, "surely he should be allowed to indulge himself in his preface."

Indulge he did, taking readers on a journey from his youth as a "conventional enough Boston-Harvard boy" to his adulthood, lingering especially over the various indignations (real and manufactured) that he suffered as a surgeon and would-be reformer. Among other vignettes documenting his misunderstood genius, he details his on-again, off-again relationship with the mighty Massachusetts General Hospital (MGH); the failure of the little ten-bed hospital nary a mile from that medical behemoth (and which he rather petulantly organized to exact revenge for wrongs, real and imagined, enacted by the MGH); his other on-again, off-again relationship with the American College of Surgeons; his habit of outraging colleagues with provocative paraphernalia—cartoons, passive-aggressive dedications, and, yes, autobiographical prefaces he was sure they would deem inappropriate. It's all here, all told with characteristic flair and perhaps just a dash of narcissism.

But apart from Codman's general audacity and Don Quixote-esque stabs at the air, what has always struck me about this preface are the reasons Codman offers to explain this odd addition to a scientific study of the shoulder. We should know him, he claims, because to know him is to know his work. Life refuses to be compartmentalized. There is continuity between life and work, after all, even if sometimes we would like to pretend, and do pretend, otherwise.

Such is certainly the case with this book, which had its start, as did my career as a historian of medicine, with a chance encounter at the University of Chicago, where I had been toiling away as a medieval historian and was knee-deep in expanding my still and forever limited skills with the Latin language. The encounter was with Alison Winter, who became my PhD adviser, my model for things to do (*do* write creatively and take chances) and not to do (*don't* use bathroom breaks as a motivating tool), and my very dear mentor and friend.

Even notwithstanding my Latin failures, medieval history wasn't in the cards for me, and Alison had the gall to take me on as a history of medicine student, for reasons I still don't know but am grateful for. She shepherded me through my PhD, through my personal foibles, through job applications, through life.

Alison was an inspirational person who was inspirationally herself at all times. The last time I visited her was at the very end of her life, when she was unable to speak but listened to me as attentively and thoughtfully as ever. When she died of a brain tumor in 2016, those who knew her, whether personally or through her works, knew they had lost something incredibly precious and rare. Others who knew her better than I did and were far dearer to her felt this loss far more keenly. And I am sure they still do, as I do. I am forever grateful. She gave me my career; she pushed me to write, think, and be more creative. I am a better person and scholar for having known her.

She was, of course, not alone among those who supported me over my years at the University of Chicago. I am grateful to Robert Richards, Jan Goldstein, and especially to Jim Sparrow and Adrian Johns for keeping up with me in the years since. I appreciate the mentorship and friendship of Sarah Igo and Cathy Gere, and I am forever grateful to Michael Allen, who was a wonderful mentor before my transition to the study of modern medicine. Thank you for never holding my poor Latinity against me.

Especially dear to me still from those years are Geoffrey Rees, the most wonderfully creative person I know, and the perennially curious and world's best and perhaps only historian-geriatrician Dan Brauner, with whom I formed a little triumvirate, injecting lashings of history into medical ethical conversation. Since then, they have both in their own way kept me going and kept me honest, each reminding me of the reasons why I like to do this work and what I hope to get out of it.

It was also over this period that I came to know the archivists and librarians who would become decade-long correspondents. Among these especially I thank Susan Rishworth and Dolores Barber at the Archives of the American College of Surgeons, who were as generous with their time as they were insightful with their advice. Also at the College, I was lucky to meet three historically minded surgeons—David Nahrwold, Peter Kernahan, and George Sheldon—who welcomed me into their fold. Susan Sacharski at the Northwestern Memorial Hospital Archives was both a witty email conversationalist and an extraordinary colleague in the navigation of the Joseph DeLee papers; Renee Ziemer at the Mayo Clinic's W. Bruce Fye Center for the History of Medicine guided me through the early years of the Mayo Clinic; and Jessica Murphy at the Special Collections and Archives at the Countway Library sent me scads of documents from the Ernest Amory Codman papers once I moved to London. Daria Wingreen at the Smithsonian, Katey Watson and the staff at the Purdue University Special Collections, where the Frank Gilbreth papers are held, and Julia Pope at the Ford Health Services Lam Archives offered vital help as the book came to completion. I am exceptionally grateful to these individuals (indeed, to all those employed behind the scenes at the institutions I visited or bothered via email for weeks or months on end) for making this book possible.

I am also grateful for the support of my more recent mentors and friends. David Edgerton and Abigail Woods brought me up professionally, and I am thankful to both of them, in different ways, for taking an interest and taking the time through many ups and downs to make sure I would thrive. I constantly appreciate the friendship of Agnes Arnold-Forster, my first PhD student and more recent co-everything-er. And I am likewise grateful to Grazia de Michele, who inspires me daily, takes no guff, and is an amazing historian and an even better friend. In my community of scholars and friends both in London and outside, I thank Adam Sutcliffe, Jon Wilson, Anna Maerker, Chris Manias, Tom Arnold-Forster, Paul Addae, Toby Green, Daniel Hadas, Jesse Olszynko-Gryn, and countless others who inspire me daily and whose conversations and interventions have made my work better in countless and critical ways.

Friends and PhD fellows-in-arms, now far-flung, still offer a constant backdrop of support. I am grateful to them all, but especially to Jen Karlin, for always fitting me in amid a schedule that is equal parts passionate clinical and intellectual work and herculean athletic feats; to Marcie Holmes, for her sharp and incisive critique on all manner of things and for walking the streets of London with me at some of my lowest points; and to Lily Huang, for constant intellectual inspiration. Deeper in my past but still constantly in my present, I thank Mary and Margaret Kowalsky and Bernard Prusak for always being just an email or a text or a phone call away, and Sarah Benioff and her family for, from the moment I met them, wholeheartedly and unquestioningly embracing me. I am also grateful to Linda and Rebecca Canino and Rachel Lavoie, who have shown me more love and taken more care than I can ever properly thank them for. They have collectively made it their business to make me their family in the deepest sense of that word.

To my family, the one I grew up with, I owe perpetual thanks as well. To my parents, Clem and Mary Kate, I owe the luxury of endless educational opportunities, constant support, and boundless love and the million joys of growing up in a house full of happiness. They didn't see this book come to fruition, but I hope that they would be proud.

My brother Denis also did not live to see this book, although in many ways its completion is his doing. Full of the most endearing (and maddening) eccentricities, he and I were of the same mind (his mind, he would always say) from early on. He walked me to kindergarten; kept me up till all hours for late-night jogging sessions—because they were better for you, he insisted—when we were teenagers; and later on in life, when we were much further apart geographically, became my daily dog-walking phone call. I hope he would be as proud of me now as I was on the occasion of his book. I am so glad that I get to celebrate with my brother Chris, a source of incredible support and perennial kindness, the cleverest of quips, and the oldest and most obscure of television theme songs, and with Jen, Eliza, and Clem.

To my current family, the family I have made, I am most grateful of all. Lola and Lexi are sources of indescribable happiness, silliness, love, and crazy, zany fun. Fox and Rizzo, and before them Larry, Cornelia, and Scrapsy, and before them Thelonious and Helga have kept me feeling loved, entertained, and well exercised for decades.

But I really owe this book to one person, the joyful, optimistic Frog to my (sometimes) gloomy, grumpy Toad—Lucas Canino. We met playing pickup soccer at the University of Chicago. I had forgotten my water bottle, so he offered me his. He has been giving me things, taking care of me, wordsmithing my sentence jumbles, listening to my ideas, generating enthusiasm and optimism for the future, producing an endless supply of ridiculous knock-knock jokes, and making my world infinitely more beautiful ever since.

Introduction

On March 1, 1915, Drs. Eugene Pool and Frederick Bancroft arrived at the Providence, Rhode Island, home of Frank and Lillian Gilbreth, the power couple behind industrial efficiency. They had been summoned there to continue an efficiency study begun several years earlier at the New York Hospital, where both Pool and Bancroft worked as surgeons. Now, standing in the Gilbreth family dining room, refashioned into a mock operating room for this "conference on the standardization of hospital practice" (figure Intro.1), they listened as Frank Gilbreth kicked off the proceedings with a diatribe. The typical operating room, he declared, was an embarrassment of inefficiency. To start, each surgeon worked with proprietary tools—all similar but *just* different enough from another surgeon's instruments as to constantly frustrate those who assisted them. And the *disorder*. Unnecessary objects and equipment lay strewn around the surgical spaces he had seen, with no evidence that their placement had been considered at all. Surgery was a circus of objects and people muddling along in what ought to have been one of the most important tasks: saving a human life.[1] And there was no agreement, Gilbreth pointed out, on what the new germ theory required of surgeons. Some surgeons wore masks, while others argued that such precautions were only necessary for those who tended to "talk over an open wound."[2] What worried him was not the inconsistent take-up of germ theory principles—something that extended across the profession and into wider society. It was the lack of any consistent procedure or standards.[3] Gilbreth was convinced that uniformity, even when arbitrarily established, led to organization, and organization led to efficient—and therefore better—surgical care.

Gilbreth's medical critique would not have been surprising to the two surgeons. Indeed, he had been dressing down medical practitioners both in person and in print for years. Fresh off his first stint in 1912 in the operating rooms of the

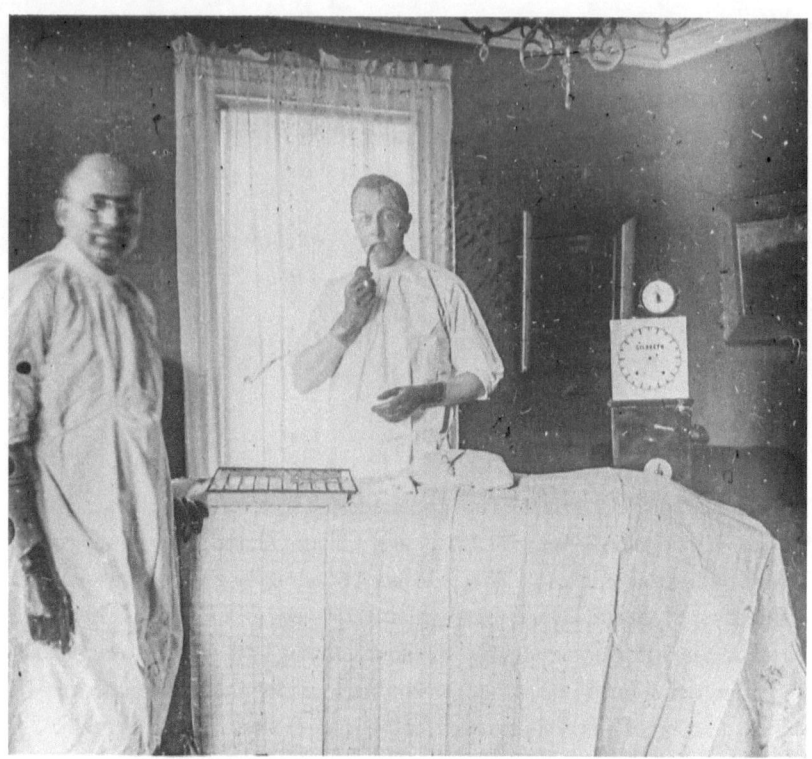

FIGURE INTRO.1. Eugene Pool (*right*) and Frederick Bancroft (*left*) taking a break from performing their surgical procedures in front of Gilbreth's cameras at the Gilbreth's Standardization Conference held at his home in Providence, Rhode Island, on March 1, 1915. Image courtesy of the Smithsonian Library and Archives, Washington, DC.

New York Hospital, where he had met Pool and Bancroft, Gilbreth told a writer at *American Magazine* that when measured against workers in other professions, surgeons were surely no better in skill than the humble dockwalloper, whose job it was to perform the leftover tasks of the shipping trade. Yet somehow, he marveled, their place in society was markedly different. While dockwallopers and bricklayers were judged as some of society's lowliest members, surgeons somehow retained their position as society's "highbrow," even though their ways of working in no way justified this level of prestige.[4] Such "caste distinctions," as he called them, were artificial, antiquated, and in need of change.[5] Indeed, in the logic of efficiency, class held little sway. There were only better and worse workers.

These charges were not unreasonable, as Pool and Bancroft knew. Though there had been major medical breakthroughs over the turn of the twentieth century—Lister's theory of asepsis, the diphtheria antitoxin, the X-ray machine—

their potential had largely been eclipsed by medicine's persistent problems. For one thing, the populist nineteenth century had given rise to a medical Babel of various sects, each with their own methods and theories about how the body worked, and each vying for patients in a crowded and chaotic medical marketplace. Meanwhile, medical education shared the problems of education more generally, insofar as it was so varied and inconstant across its different institutional settings that it was impossible to tell what a medical student actually needed to know in order to be an effective practitioner. Most hospitals were dismal affairs—sometimes dirty, always inefficient. And the process of codifying and organizing knowledge of symptoms, diseases, and treatments for illness and injury, which began in the nineteenth century, was still slow.[6] This was no small thing, since without a common nomenclature, even sharing information about a disease was a tricky business. Like surgical tools, the diagnosis and treatment of pathologies depended largely on the experience and preferences of each individual practitioner.

To Pool and Bancroft, the right solution to this medical malaise—the solution that had brought them on this pilgrimage to Providence—lay in efficiency study.[7] And they were not alone in this belief. In fact, as Gilbreth informed a meeting of efficiency experts, the Gilbreths "ha[d] not met a single doctor in our travels who has opposed us; we . . . had the finest cooperation of nurses, and from every trustee whom we have met."[8] Like his famous contemporary and erstwhile mentor Frederick Winslow Taylor, Gilbreth was best known for his interventions in factories, where he applied the standardizing and rationalizing instruments of efficiency study to industrial workers and their labor. But he was also no stranger to medicine, often boasting that his work on surgery and in hospitals, undertaken with his wife Lillian (his business partner, coauthor, and prominent industrial psychologist) had taken him "from Maine to California inclusive, through the rivers of Quebec and Toronto" and "as far north as Stockholm and as far south as Italy." It was a geographic breadth of experience that led the Gilbreths to one damning conclusion: "The doctors," he told a mixed meeting of efficiency experts and medical practitioners in 1916, "are awful." And though he had "not lost all confidence in mankind," Frank Gilbreth said, his experience of medical labor and of the state of the hospitals in the United States was anything but reassuring.[9]

Happily, Gilbreth did see some points of light scattered across the professional darkness. In this speech before the Taylor Society, he cited at least a hundred fifty practitioners who had actively "co-operated with him" in these studies, though he confined himself in that speech to dropping a few big names. Though it is unclear if or when he had met them, Gilbreth talked about

William and Charles Mayo, whose work in efficiency was so well known that Gilbreth said he felt it hardly necessary to discuss it. He gave a shout-out to Pool and Bancroft and a nod to Ernest Amory Codman, the famously snappish surgeon and efficiency guru whose outlandish efforts to reform the profession had earned him a real reputation in the East Coast medical world.

Then there was the obstetrician Robert Latou Dickinson, "for whom," Gilbreth told those gathered to hear his speech, "he had the highest admiration," even though he was, Gilbreth privately confided in Pool and Bancroft, "ridiculous" when it came to matters of efficiency.[10] And of course he could not forget, he noted, the hospital superintendent and efficiency enthusiast Thomas Howell, who had facilitated his studies at the New York Hospital.

Clearly, Frank Gilbreth loved to grandstand, but his swagger was not without substance. His name was certainly a respected one to many medical practitioners and administrators with a modernizing bent. He was known to the medical heavyweight Sigismund S. Goldwater, a hospital superintendent and editor of the efficiency-suffused journal, the *Modern Hospital*, which dedicated its inaugural issue in 1913 to efficient hospital management, design, and organization. And he was familiar to John Hornsby, another *Modern Hospital* editor and writer of the popular "Items in Hospital Efficiency" column in the journal. Indeed, there is good reason to think that the Gilbreths rubbed elbows with all the major figures in this medical efficiency moment. Even the educational reformer Abraham Flexner, best known for his audit and standardization of American and Canadian medical schools, knew their work well enough to comment on the likelihood of success for a proposed collaboration with Dickinson in 1914. It would have been hard for him not to: Gilbreth proselytized his medical efficiency work as widely as he could, welcoming the possibility of speaking at any venue that would have him and publishing multiple discussions of the value of medical efficiency in the medical and lay literature.

Though they are both associated today almost exclusively with industry, both the Gilbreths and—more importantly—efficiency made a pronounced splash in early twentieth-century medicine. And it was no mere dalliance. Efficiency principles were translated directly to measures like the standardization of medical education, surgeons, hospitals, diseases, and therapies. They were also integral to the developing logic of medical mores—namely, that rationalized processing made a "good" product, and that good medical products should be replicable and disseminable. And this in turn was what medical organizations sold to the public: not an *effective* set of treatments or therapies necessarily, though they might also be that, but a set of *standard* therapies and the promise of *thorough* processing. What "modern" medicine could uniquely offer was efficiency.

Though the reach and breadth of medical efficiency was undoubtedly widespread and its implications for medicine profound (in both epistemological and material ways), medical efficiency has never been a hot topic for historians of medicine. It has received particularly short shrift despite—or perhaps because of—Frank's explicit, rather showy and well-publicized forays into medicine. This despite the fact that, as Flexner observed, the sheer ubiquity of efficiency in this period made ridiculous the supposition that it would not be an actor in every educational discussion, including medicine.[11] Not only was medicine subject to the same cultural pressures as other parts of American life, it also explicitly sought out the kind of intervention that efficiency could provide. So where has medical efficiency gone? And what was its story?

Though in many ways the reinstatement of efficiency that this book undertakes seems straightforward—filling the gaps, as one does, in the historical record—it accomplishes much more than that. For one thing, it recaptures a key mechanism of medicine's modernization—one that we continue, in the public sphere, to chalk up to a rather vaguely constituted but firmly held idea of scientific and technological innovation. In their own time, medical efficiency enthusiasts rejected this view. Instead, they saw efficiency as the fundamental catalyst of medical modernization—the entity that energized preexisting pushes to order medicine in epistemological, bureaucratic, and professional terms and added to them the modernist values of the early twentieth century.[12] And though its proponents continued to maintain that medicine was "scientific" and therefore modern, it is clear that they understood efficiency to be an essential part of their science, one that demanded the "systematic . . . accumulation of data, the framing of hypotheses, and the checking up of results."[13] It was the "science" of efficiency that made medicine modern, and this has had underrecognized but great significance across both the history and contemporary of American medicine.

Of course, there *is* more to medicine than just the management of information, and medical efficiency experts in the early twentieth century thought so, too. Their adoption of efficiency was only partly predicated on the real, quantifiable improvements to organization that medical efficiency could deliver. It also carried a more ephemeral set of qualities and characteristics that held for them the promise of something even greater.

Here, the specifics of medical efficiency meet the larger history of efficiency in the United States, revealing a new story. Unlike the history of industrial efficiency in the main, where individuals like Taylor and Henry Ford along with businesses like the Ford Motor Company, Standard Oil, and US Steel dominate both the archive and the narrative, medical efficiency has featured a more diffuse array of actors, organizations, and activities.[14] And perhaps because of their elevated medical "caste," as Gilbreth put it, their voices have been preserved in the archive.[15] Of course, we cannot know everything that the rank and file of medical practitioners experienced, since only medicine's louder and more powerful voices had their words recorded and their records kept for posterity, but the dynamic views and discussions among even these highbrow practitioners still shed light on the intrinsic ambivalences of efficiency, in theory as in practice. For one thing, it shows a remarkable willingness among practitioners to align themselves and their work with the world of the factory floor.

What results is a story that shifts efficiency's near singular significance as the de-skilling source of monopoly capitalism into a rather more dynamic if at times utterly contradictory experiment in American democracy. Ida Tarbell, who was famous for her muckraking exposé of the monopolistic and antidemocratic activities of Standard Oil, differentiated monopoly from efficiency, explaining in 1917 that efficiency done right was not "in conflict with democracy" but "on the contrary . . . ha[d] come as a sympathetic handmaiden of democracy, showing her how she can help men to develop themselves along the line of their inner call."[16]

Though a dramatic story in its own right, especially for the tension between efficiency as an oppressive, disciplining force, on one hand, and a democratic, creative principle on the other, the reappraisal of efficiency also raises questions about its relation to the story that efficiency has been most specifically tied to—namely, the history of modern capitalism.

Historiographical Considerations

The general sidelining of Gilbreth's quest to bring efficiency to medicine is representative of the absence of efficiency more broadly in the stories we tell about medicine's modernization over the early twentieth century. Because neither of the Gilbreths were medical practitioners (despite Frank's insistence that his own knowledge of medicine was substantial, not least because of the many children he had "chaperoned . . . into the world"), their placement outside the medical profession has looked to some as though they lacked the standing to seriously inspire any reform in medicine's hierarchical and closed workplace. Seemingly, the highbrow status of the surgeons and medical practitioners that Gilbreth had been so keen to bring down gave these practitioners no reason to listen to the Gilbreths or to yield to their efficiency interventions.[17]

The historical record does not support this view. But the historiographical one at least explains it. The marginalization of efforts like the Gilbreths' has at least something to do with the way in which the lessons of power were thought to be differently manifested in the history of medicine compared with business and industry.

Though with conceptual origins that ran all the way back to the 1930s, the new social history of medicine of the 1970s and 1980s saw power as the operative structure of medicine's twentieth-century history. This in large part arose from the milieu created by anti-institutional figures like Ivan Illich, Thomas McKeown, and Archie Cochrane, whose radically different takes on medicine nonetheless rested on the relatively common thread: that medicine had never been—or at least in McKeown's softened view, had not until recently been—actually *effective*.[18] Though Illich was by far the most extreme of the bunch, not least for his belief that medicine was actively harmful to human health, even the most conservative of these commentators agreed with this basic premise. Their supporting evidence lay in charts that showed the relative powerlessness of vaccines in the wake of rising and falling infectious disease over decades; in the absence of progress in the fight against cancer; and in the arrival of the major new health catastrophe, AIDS.

This view that medicine was not especially effective raised a pressing question: how had medicine acquired such comprehensive cultural and political control if it fundamentally lacked the clinical and scientific efficacy on which that power had presumptively stood? The answer for many was professionalization, and it was one that built medicine back into the language of capitalism.[19] For those like Paul Starr, the keen-eyed historical sociologist, it was taken for granted that the transformation of medicine from a small-scale set of disunified and locally specific operations to the cultural and political behemoth it became had to have been the result of a social—not clinical—transformation.[20]

Efficiency was a poor fit for this new narrative. In its industrial contexts, it was being rediscovered and then positioned into a different version of power acquisition—through capitalist integration—that conflicted with medicine's own. The reading of figures like Frederick Winslow Taylor, the "father of scientific management," and Henry Ford centered on the way in which the rationalization of work denied both agency and subjectivity to workers. With these men blazing the trail, the efficiency "managerial class" shut out the voices and expertise of workers, replacing them with arbitrary and bureaucratic forms of control—all in service to the "almighty dollar" and manifested in the monopolistic successes of individuals like Andrew Carnegie and John D. Rockefeller, whose fortunes were built on the back of the working class. Though this view of industrial efficiency has since been increasingly nuanced and even contested within the academic literature, it is nonetheless still commonplace to assume that Taylorism, Fordism, or scientific management (or any of the other monikers used to designate industrial efficiency) embodied, as Harry Braverman famously put it, capitalist production. It would not go too far to say, then, that to many scholars, Taylorism not only opened the door to the monopoly capitalism of the early twentieth century, it *was* monopoly capitalism at the small or local scale.[21]

Intuitively, where efficiency is about the exertion of power over workers, the imposition of efficiency study onto medical workers, with its implicit threat of presenting an external, industrially inflected managerial class, runs up against the story of professionalization, where authority was acquired by medicine and from within. From that perspective, the methods of efficiency study projects like Gilbreth's, especially as they functioned in the literature as methods for the acquisition of power, did not look like they could have a place in medicine *until* they were appropriated into the apparatus of medicine's power acquisition project. At that point, Flexner's efficiency-suffused study of medical education, which many assert he took up at the behest of the American Medical Association (AMA), together with the standardization efforts of large medical organizations (especially the AMA, the American College of Surgeons, and the American Hospital Association) and the actions of medicine's monopolistic cabal (known as "organized medicine"), were all seen as playing a role in how medical power was acquired by and for medicine.[22]

Perhaps because of these poorly meshing narratives, much historical literature simply offers up medical efficiency as a failed endeavor or historical outtake: the phenomenon that could have succeeded—but didn't—in preventing the coming capitalism of the medical marketplace.[23] There have since been critical additions, including the study of standards in the American context and even scientific management and industrial efficiency in medicine outside of it.[24] None of these, though, have been able to capture the full picture of medical efficiency, which extended far beyond its practical application.

One finds some initial grist for this mill in the scholarly argument about the meaning and scope of industrial efficiency. Some have argued that industrial efficiency interventions were limited in scope and impact and thus could never have achieved the characteristic widespread de-skilling they were supposed to have enabled in the name of monopoly capitalism. Others have shot back that industrial efficiency was more of a movement than a set of specific practices, so that even if it was limited in practice, it marked the transformative change in the ideology of labor that made capitalism.[25]

But the problem is that in the American context at least, efficiency was certainly not limited to industrial contexts. Nor was it only in medicine. It was *everywhere*. Indeed, between 1910, when Louis Brandeis brought the term "scientific management" to the attention of the public with his claim, printed in the newspapers, that it could save the railroads "one million dollars a day," and 1929, when the rude awakening of the Great Depression remade efficiency into public enemy number one, efficiency played a large part—some might say an integral part—in American life.[26] As Samuel Haber's classic work on the subject described, efficiency was so ubiquitous and so well regarded over this period that to say that something was "efficient" was just about the highest praise possible.[27]

This was the era of efficiency in government, with departments dedicated to improving government function by reducing waste, and in the conservation movement, where it helped to build a formula for the more responsible use of flora and fauna.[28] It was efficiency that led Melville Dewey to create his eponymous system for organizing, standardizing, and streamlining American libraries (in campaigning tirelessly to reform the inefficiencies of English spelling, Dewey even streamlined his own name, for a while operating under the sobriquet "Melvil Dui").[29] Meanwhile, Lillian Gilbreth was introducing efficiency to the domestic sphere, producing the modern kitchen with its cabinets above and below and ergonomic worktops along with other space- and step-saving solutions.[30]

The Gilbreths applied their gospel everywhere, often carrying out work in front of large crowds. They turned their attention to sports, studying rowing, golf, and, on one bright sunny spring day in 1913, baseball. On the very last day of May, the roughly twenty thousand who turned up to watch the New York Giants play the Philadelphia Phillies at the Polo Grounds were given the unexpected pregame pleasure of witnessing the Gilbreths perform a showy master class in efficiency study that promised to advantage the base stealer and pitcher alike (figure Intro.2).[31]

Efficiency was also something people could personalize. From 1914 to 1918, Edward Purinton, a self-appointed personal efficiency expert and director of the *Independent*'s efficiency service, offered life advice in the magazine's "Efficiency Question Box" section for readers seeking spiritual and material uplift from efficiency. Purinton was prolific, with a purview that covered just about everything, from the best way to vacation (do whatever is the most opposite of one's work) to the best way to discover one's true passion.[32]

And efficiency could be found woven through contemporary literature. Edith Wharton, marking the final days of the efficiency craze in 1927, named the protagonist in her novel *Twilight Sleep* Pauline Manford (man-Ford). The character was a woman so obsessed with efficiency and the productivity it enabled that she wanted to standardize the emotional vagaries right out of the human heart, replacing it with an organ where function singularly followed its form.[33]

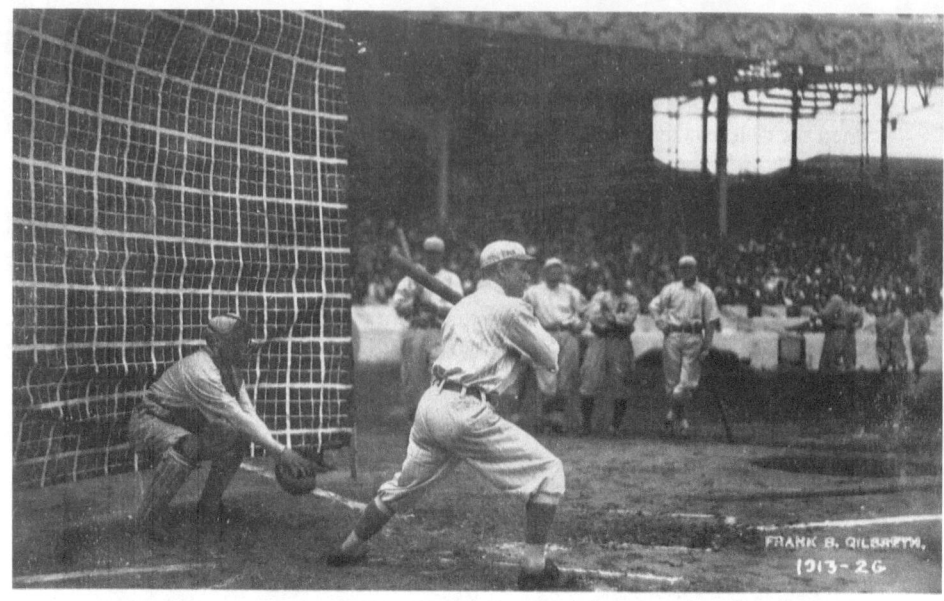

FIGURE INTRO.2. Larry Doyle of the New York Giants is at bat to take part in Gilbreth's efficiency studies of baseball, held during the pregame of a Giants versus Philadelphia Phillies game on May 31, 1913. The *New York Tribune* ran the photo two weeks later, noting that "according to the pictorial record in this case, the swing of the batter's bat until it struck the ball occupied .042 of a second." Image courtesy of the Frank and Lillian Gilbreth Library of Management Research and Professional Papers, Purdue University Libraries Archives and Special Collections, West Lafayette, Indiana.

Whether sidelined as the more nefarious (because more insidious) signs of efficiency's total control over American politics and culture or dismissed as amusing cultural side effects of what was squarely an industrial story, these many colorful iterations of efficiency have been given short shrift. But they point to the malleability of efficiency as a concept and its persistence as a method that, just as it certainly enacted an autocratic logic in the factory, was simultaneously enacting a thoroughly democratic logic in public life.[34] It is this counterintuitive mix of explicitly democratic, even populist, theoretical underpinnings and equally explicit antidemocratic, monopolistic tendencies that come together in medical efficiency.[35]

This tension has already come out in a few studies of the Gilbreths, whose more outlandish displays of efficiency and conspicuous quest for egalitarianism helped single out their efforts historically.[36] Indeed, it was not exceptional for Gilbreth to insist, as he did in the pages of the *American Magazine*, that surgery was just another form of manual labor that any dockwalloper properly trained could do. Less an explicit takedown of medical practice (though it was also that), the article registered efficiency's well-known egalitarian values and its potential for social mobility.[37] More recent studies that take a closer look at Fordism find similar tensions. Important distinctions might be made, for example, between the personal beliefs and policies of Henry Ford and the conceptual system of Fordism that ultimately bore his name. Stefan Link makes a convincing case for the rethinking of Ford's own relationship with work and workers, in part by addressing head on the ambivalence of Ford's views and the views that grew around him into "Fordism."[38]

Indeed, any account of medical efficiency must grapple with these tensions. While the story here is partly about the science of medicine that efficiency made, it is also and sometimes more prominently about the struggle to make medicine a modern entity, insofar as it was both egalitarian and democratic and also standard-driven and tightly codified.

In this sense, *The Product of Medicine* is chiefly concerned with telling the story of medical efficiency as one of modernization extending from the origins of efficiency in the factory, across American political, cultural, and economic life, and into medicine. Hardly just a monolithic power acquisition process, efficiency lent medicine a form, a set of functions, and a logic that spelled out what seem now to be efficiency's counterintuitive, even sometimes apparently mutually exclusive, goals and aims—on the one hand, autocracy and monopoly; on the other, liberation and social mobility.

At the same time, this work also creates an opportunity to see, through the far more visible lens of medical efficiency, how efficiency was constituted. And where efficiency is viewed as having critical importance for understanding the shape and scope of industrial capitalism, it sheds light too on how early twentieth-century figures understood the potential of efficiency to create the modern democracy they hoped the United States would become.

At least for some. Medical efficiency, and efficiency more broadly, was primarily a white preoccupation focused most often on the structuring and needs of the growing middle class. It was a movement aimed at those *Collier's* journalist Bruce Barton referred to as the "silent majority," who "were neither radicals nor reactionaries" but "middle of the road folks who own their own homes and work hard."[39] Where race did enter into early twentieth-century discussions, it is often explicitly parenthetical: the othered discussion and debates that were happening outside efficiency spaces proper.

The book traces the contours of this exclusion, particularly by noticing where and, perhaps more importantly, *how* it is performed. There is the "blink and you'll miss it" discussion of the Black medical schools slotted into the very last pages of Flexner's famous report; the characteristically contradictory understanding of race and efficiency in the Ford "empire"; and the explicit concerns of the National Medical Association (NMA), the Black physicians organization, over the segregationist implications of the medical efficiency fixes made at the American College of Surgeons.[40] Commenting on hospital standardization efforts during the 1920s, the president of the NMA noted crucially that it wasn't necessarily that standardizing organizations intentionally aimed to hurt the Black medical community. It was that "they had not considered us at all."[41]

There is an obvious point here: efficiency and its attendant values were in this way explicitly emblematic of the particular racism of the early twentieth century. Efficiency in these contexts was emptied of its content as a vehicle for considerations of the demands of American democracy and ceased to concern either of its conceptual extremes: egalitarianism, on the one hand, and autocracy on the other. Instead, it became yet another weapon in an already enormous social arsenal dedicated, whether intentionally or not, to segregation and exclusion. Though in ways more complex than they seem at first blush, efficiency created and to some degree also policed both implicit and explicit racial lines within medicine. Here, then, the book offers glimpses of the institutionalization of racism within medicine and the navigation of these limits within Black medical organizations over the period in which medicine became modern.

Structure

The Product of Medicine is organized thematically to capture medical efficiency in its many registers and functions over its heyday—the first half of the twentieth century. Chapter 1 examines some of the essential material gains that efficiency brought to medicine. With an emphasis on the establishment of medical products, as these were being reimagined by the efficiency logic of the day, it opens with the failure of medical practitioners to reach a conclusion on what it was that medicine produced. This looks now like an existential concern about medical effectiveness. In fact, the determination of a product was the starting point of the efficiency method. Essential to efficiency study was the designation of a product. Only once this was established could attendant processes be rationalized in pursuit of improving efficiency.

For their obvious kinship with industrial processes, insofar as each supplied a product at the end of a process, digestion and childbirth were natural targets for efficiency interventions. But like industrial processes, questions about how best to relate the process by which a product was made to the product itself guided considerations of both. The chapter specifically examines the turn of attention to the rationalization of process that came increasingly to guide ideas about what good childbirth looked like and what best digestive practices required of an eater. But this was not a problem internal only to the human body, as the chapter demonstrates via discussion of the process-oriented, assembly-line method of care at the very successful and already dearly beloved Mayo Clinic.

Chapter 2 moves into the meeting of industrial mores and medical values that took place at the Henry Ford Hospital. Billed in its own time as an institution that would import and apply Ford's assembly-line practices to medicine, the chapter describes the ways in which the Ford Hospital, in its most modern qualities, was distinctly *un*-Fordist. That is, its modernizing principles were borrowed largely from the other major modern hospitals of the day—those that had already adopted efficiency as their watchword in myriad ways. The single caveat to this Fordist story, arguably the single way in which the Ford Hospital was really a "Ford product," was in the heady mix of efficiency and democracy, of control and mobility, that guided Ford's insistence on charging consumers who arrived at the hospital a flat rate: a logic that sprang directly from what is now his rather counterfactual insistence that capitalism, when done right, would foster meaningful social uplift.

Chapters 3 and 4 build on this counterfactual, delving into two of the most prominent examples of medical standardization, first at the American College of Surgeons and then in the hands of medicine's best-known standardizer, Abraham Flexner and his (in)famous report for the Carnegie Foundation on the state of medical education and the prospects for its repair.

The third chapter focuses on the hospital standardization effort of the American College of Surgeons. It traces the efficiency logic that led from a purely populist notion of standardization—where standards were adopted because of their popular appeal—to a system that, to its proponents at least, avoided both the chaos of populism *and* the rigidity that made efficiency autocratic, arriving at a manifestation of standardization that seemed therefore properly democratic.

These competing ideologies were also at the heart of Flexner's study and subsequent attempts to standardize medical education, which is taken up in chapter 4. Though generally read as an instrument of medical professionalization, Flexner's body of work in educational reform attests to his belief—however naïve—in efficiency's power to both maintain and develop educational egalitarianism. In many ways, the project failed, yielding instead to a far more capitalist, exclusionary logic that parsed the medical world in ways that Flexner seemed not to anticipate. But in his attempts nonetheless to maintain efficiency's competing demands, and in his general failure to do so, we catch a first glimpse of the way efficiency begot or became capitalism: not as the thing it was always meant to be, but as the thing that it ineluctably became when the small scale of efficiency study hit the large scale of racist, classist, and sexist politics and culture in the United States. Although these issues received their fullest airing at the time in the context of the so-called poor boy that critics claimed would always be on the outside of Flexner's reforms, the chapter ends with a fuller consideration of where these standardization attempts left Black students of medicine.

Chapter 5 returns to the American College of Surgeons to consider its attempts to "sell" its standard hospital across the country. In contrast to the Flexnerian outcome, the College continued to manage its delicate balance of autocratic method and egalitarian ethos. In the construction of a market for the standard hospital—the College could not survive, it realized, without one—the ACS managed always to stop just short of the out-of-bounds capitalism that Flexner's standardizing efforts had come to embody and that its contemporary, the AMA, seemed fully to embrace. The arc of the story will not be unfamiliar to those who know of the work of other medical organizations of the period that were "selling" health with all the verve that patent medicine operators had deployed to sell their tonics. The chapter, however, turns both on the uniqueness of the College's product—"standard" and *therefore* modern medicine—and on the College's surprising success as a standardizing body.

The book closes with a well-known moment in medicine's history in the United States: the events leading up to and around the prosecution of the AMA as a monopoly. In this way, chapter 6 marks the end of the efficiency movement, which was ushered out by the Depression and the shifting mores of medicine, away from the moorings in efficiency and toward the power-acquisition processes that historians have more generally described. But this is still not all there is to say. For even as medicine became more monolithic as an industry itself, it also became more polarized, resolving the tensions intrinsic to efficiency into the two extrinsic poles of modern medicine that are still with us now: as a powerful and nefarious medicalizing behemoth, on the one hand, and a beneficent and effective service for those who need it, on the other.

Though this book is embedded in the twentieth-century medical efficiency moment, I hope it also helps reconceptualize where we are right now. *The Product of Medicine* softens what has been a rather narrowed vision of medicine's twentieth-century history as first a story about power acquisition. And though the book also follows in some part from the understanding that modern medicine, like nearly all places of work in this period, moved with the prevailing winds of industrial capitalism, it shows that the terms and obligations of these prevailing winds are not as clear as we have perhaps thought. Medical attempts to designate an essential identity for modern medicine may have begun with familiar capitalist questions about how to produce a marketable product, how to get people to buy it, and how to get them to *need* it. But medicine was not only on a quest to become economically legible via the establishment of a monopoly. Just as crucial was the achievement of its cultural legibility as a legitimately democratic, legitimately modern, and in that sense legitimately useful industry.

In our own time, perhaps this book will spur a reconsideration of how we think about what medicine has meant or what it can mean. Indeed, this work is quietly invested in introducing how this history of medicine might change our relationship to health care and its reform today. One of the difficulties attendant in writing medical history is how conspiratorial it can seem from the outside: the AMA as medical history's nefarious actor, hell-bent on avoiding a federal plan of health care provision, is not even six degrees removed from the conspiracy-laced notion that Bill Gates wants to plant microchips in our bodies with the COVID-19 vaccine. So polarized are our discussions about medicine that the primary response is the same glossy, superficial narrative that thinking in terms of a "social transformation" went to such lengths to displace: that medicine achieved its vaunted cultural position by dint of effective therapies, the miracles, the lifesaving practices, the scientific progress that have made it the beneficent and lifesaving venture it is today.

In a response to Christy Ford Chapin's prompt to think about what the intertwining histories of medicine and capitalism might yield, the eminent historian of medicine Nancy Tomes observes that understanding the interplay of medicine with the larger world around it, including capitalism, gives us a chance to "'pop the hood and look inside'" to see in greater detail the workings of medicine and industry in the early part of the twentieth century.[42] This is indeed what she has done in her own books on the transformation of medicine in the context of capitalism. And it is what this book also aims to do—to offer a new historical perspective on this tumultuous period in hopes that this particular effort to "look under the hood" reminds us that there is a wide and broad analytic space between scientific positivism and conspiracy. And that is where medicine makes its home.

1

The Product

The mother is the factory, and by education and care she can be made more efficient in the art of motherhood.—GRANTLY DICK-READ, *Childbirth without Fear*, 1942

In May 1913, at a gathering of the Philadelphia County Medical Society, the surgeon and medical efficiency enthusiast Ernest Amory Codman put a challenge to the assembled doctors. "I imagine that it's not difficult," he preambled, "to render an exact account of the product of a factory. So many dozen tin cans, cakes of soap, toothpicks, or pickled pigs' feet are readily figured up." But what, he asked, "are the products of a hospital?" As a prompt, he provided a chart that he had created showing various by-products of the Massachusetts General Hospital (115 medical and surgical papers, 54 nurses graduated, etc.), as well as intake statistics (6,896 patients treated, with a 16-day average stay). These things could be tabulated and studied, he declared, but the actual end-result of a hospital remained an unknown quantity. The floor was then opened up for discussion, but the medical society failed to reach a consensus that day—Philadelphia's physicians had no ready answer for what exactly a hospital produced.[1]

A few years later, there was still no agreement when other practitioners were similarly queried by the industrial efficiency expert Frank Gilbreth. When the doctors seemed to reject his proposed product—"happiness minutes," a measurement that he had adopted in his factory work—Gilbreth reassured them that the product they chose did not actually matter as long as they decided on *something*. Without a defined product, a hospital could not define its processes, let alone improve them. What's more, without a *uniform* product, one that could be widely agreed on, medicine would be condemned to chaos, leaving doctors to offer a ragbag of various services that would confuse consumers with its variable and inconsistent claims.[2]

The story of what American medicine came to produce over the following decades, and how that product helped transform it into the force that it is today, has been told before. As Paul Starr demonstrated in his classic work on the subject, medicine underwent a social transformation in the first few decades of the twentieth century, from a disparate and disorganized collection of practitioners into a "sovereign profession" and then into a "vast industry" that followed neatly and irrevocably thereon.[3] This was, essentially, the story of how medicine became a capitalist enterprise. In this reading, any search for a product was the essential element of a nascent business plan—a plan that lay the groundwork for the full-scale professional reorganization to soon follow. "To gain the trust that the practice of medicine requires," Starr wrote, "physicians had to assure the public of the reliability of their product." And this "standardized product," in turn, Starr wrote, "require[d] a standardized profession."[4]

But as much as histories like Starr's have helped to make sense of modern medicine's ascent to cultural supremacy in the United States, the medical efficiency adherents who were proposing these product-based fixes had goals that were meaningfully different from that of setting the stage for medicine's marriage with capitalism. Codman, for example, saw in the absence of a product the core reason that medicine lacked any accountability to its patients—without a product, there was no way to measure the quality or effectiveness of medical practitioners. Some of this was most certainly personal. Though Codman ascribed to the view that products were necessary for what they could yield about process, he was also driven in his work by the vision of his own colleagues at the storied Massachusetts General Hospital—those he said had earned their positions by "nepotism, pull and politics"—finally having their comeuppance. When measured against a common product that ran across the profession, they would surely be outed as the poor practitioners Codman considered them to be.[5]

For most efficiency experts, though, the significance of a product lay not in its potential to introduce accountability but rather in its utility for evaluating the processes that produced it. As Gilbreth affirmed to his medical audiences (and Starr's own narrative hinted), there was a vital and complex relationship between product and process. This was a different beast entirely from the one described in the grand narrative of capitalism's overtaking of medicine. In that story, the crux of this relationship hangs on the notion that in medicine—as in factories—the presumptive "product" was whatever a factory produced, marketed, and sold. Paired with this notion was an equally reductive view of efficiency as a straightforward rationalization of workers, as though they too were simply machine parts whose sole role was to facilitate the unrelenting and always increasing pace of production.[6]

In medicine, the definition of product was more usefully opaque. Gilbreth's assertion that "happiness minutes" might be the right product in medicine had little to do with what he thought medicine's consumers would actually consume. Indeed, these minutes, which roughly measured the amount of time the workers in any department were "happy," were borrowed from a study of fatigue that Frank and his wife, Lillian Gilbreth, had undertaken previously.[7] And though fatigue study was of course distally related to productivity—tired workers were not, after all, productive workers, so understanding the science of "rest" was critical to the study of work—the instrumentalized, abstracted nature of this product-process nexus was a key part of efficiency methodology more broadly that existed independently from its most often-invoked context of industrial capitalism. Indeed, this reading is bolstered by Gilbreth's follow-up suggestion to his medical audiences that if they did not want to choose happiness minutes, they could, in fact, choose something else. Anything else. As long as they could agree on it. The point was only to select a product—*any* product. Without a product as the destination, the process—the journey to this destination—could not be effectively evaluated.

The focus efficiency experts placed on the product-process nexus inverts the usual relationship we presume between product and process, where a preselected product determines the shape and focus of its process. In efficiency study, and especially medical efficiency study, process held primacy, and products were determined not because they were desirable in their own right but for their instrumental value in tweaking the process they measured.

Probably one of the best-known examples of this logic in action comes in the efficiency activities of the Ford Motor Company in its production of the Model T, the final shape and form of which was determined not by a consumer-driven demand for a particular car but by a total commitment to the complete rationalization of its production process. For egalitarian reasons, Ford wanted to drive down prices and make the car affordable to those outside the upper class to whom most automobiles had been marketed. Unlike other car manufacturers, who selected cars that they thought buyers would want and set about building them, Ford allowed the total rationalization of processes to determine the final shape and form of his Model T. The wildly popular result was a product that was essentially the manifestation of the process that had created it. No frills, total uniformity, and with parts that were therefore totally interchangeable.[8]

This chapter traces the shifting emphases in this relationship across different contexts. It begins with examples that consider the meeting of this efficiency-suffused formulation of product-process logic with the preexisting understanding of the body-as-machine that guided much of the logic of conventional medical practice. It then examines how process slowly came to supersede any notion of products as important or useful in their own right. The chapter ends with this relationship as it stood at the time of the Ford Factory, where the very value of medical products—at what was possibly Ford's heavyweight equivalent in medicine, the Mayo Clinic—was understood explicitly and entirely in terms of the qualities of its processing.

In a way, the logic of product-process is quite a belabored one: one might, after all, and probably more reasonably, replace this language of product and process with terms such as "goals" or "aims" instead. In certain senses, though, the belaboring was exactly the point. The very premise of efficiency study, emphasized particularly in critical views of the activities of efficiency experts, was the formalization of knowledge structures, specifically to displace what was called, in the factory, the "rule of thumb" knowledge that workers had uniquely acquired by their own experience and insight.

Critical to the efficiency movement more broadly, then, was the replacement of this kind of knowledge with one instead packaged in the more formalized language of science, with its attendant claims to objectivity.[9] Though often glossed *merely* as a way to disempower workers or, in medical contexts, to disempower patients, in fact the formalization of language that product-process obligated was useful in its own right. And in many senses, this is precisely what the product-process logic occasioned: on the one hand, a clearly duplicitous attempt to grab power through the formalization of bias into the language of objectivity, and on the other, a clear attempt to structure study and formulate intervention along rationalized lines.[10]

Body Processes

By the early twentieth century, the notion that the body functioned as a machine was quite an old one. As Anson Rabinbach described in his seminal study *The Human Motor*, the body-as-machine analogy began with Descartes, traveled through adherents to the physiologic "mechanical" body of the eighteenth century, and arrived in the nineteenth century as a body that acted and reacted as motors also did, marking out the space for the fatigue studies that Gilbreth and others ported into their efficiency work.[11] Over the nineteenth century, this view of the body helped to catalyze what Charles Rosenberg called a "therapeutic revolution," which shifted the view of disease from one predicated on the idiosyncrasy of individual bodies, with thus no uniformity across bodies or its parts, to one that rested on the notion that bodies were all uniform: the malfunctions of one body were, then, of a piece with the expectable malfunctions of all bodies.[12]

In the early twentieth century, this view shifted slightly to reflect a more explicitly efficiency-suffused permutation of the body-as-machine, in which the body became the "symbolic object of efficient management and regulation" in myriad ways.[13] And though over this period, much discussion turned on questions of workers' rights in the new regime of hyperproductivity (a particular feature in the context of ever-increasing labor unrest over the 1910s and 1920s), efficiency's utilitarian logic of process-product held attraction to medicine, not least because of the explanatory power that this logic seemed to hold for the exploration and therapeutic manipulation of otherwise autonomous body processes.[14]

One of these was digestion. Though we know him better for other reasons today, at the turn of the century, John Harvey Kellogg was among the best-known proponents of this product-process logic in the digestive arena. Starting with his book *The Stomach*, the surgeon and cereal magnate (with brother Will Keith) put forward the view that the stomach played such an essential role in health that the body ought to be considered as a "stomach with various organs appended."[15] And though his ideas certainly owed much to earlier nineteenth-century theories about the relationship between the health of the gastrointestinal tract and the body, Kellogg tested and refined his ideas of digestive efficiency over decades of work in his own human laboratory: the Battle Creek Sanitarium in Michigan. Though his facility also offered hydro-, electro-, photo-, and other popular types of "wellness" therapy, no patients who sought relief at the "san" from a spectrum of illnesses and complaints could avoid Kellogg's intensive focus on the tracking and reform of their digestive system and dietary habits.[16]

There was also Horace Fletcher, known to his loyal following as the "Great Masticator." As colorful as Kellogg but less well remembered, Fletcher charged his acolytes to chew any solid food until it was rendered liquid (and then chew liquids until they were more liquid) before swallowing. This meal-prolonging process, dubbed "Fletcherization," was thought to bestow healing on the ill and protection to the healthy explicitly by reestablishing the mouth as a vital locus of food *processing*. In Fletcher's view, this achieved a lightening of the processing load on the rest of the system and ensured that food made a smoother and faster trip through and out of the body.[17]

Both digestive doyens espoused the view that digestion was a process in need of manipulation, but they differed on the significance of the product that digestion produced. For Fletcher, "digestive ash," as he politely called feces, was not a real product but rather an indicator of waste. True to the efficiency credo of the day, he believed that maximizing the efficiency of the system should reduce this waste, ideally to zero. Fletcher thus viewed digestive ash as problematic for its very presence, for it signaled the inefficiency of the processes within it.[18] Under the logic that the only part of the process that a person could control was the chewing, the rest being the responsibility of the body itself, Fletcher's solution to this problem was to advise that anything that could not be liquefied in the mouth ought best be unceremoniously "returned to the plate," in order to avoid forcing the digestive system to expend energy on creating what would be, after all, only waste products.

Kellogg agreed with Fletcher's view that digestive processing was of paramount importance, but he broke with the Great Masticator, whom he dismissed as a food faddist in part because of the reductiveness of his logic, on the value of what Kellogg preferred to call, more bluntly, "bowel movements."[19] Kellogg did not see these products as mere waste, not least because this label denied the value that bowel movements held to describe the process happening within. Instead, the more sophisticated Kellogg saw bowel movements as essential products quite in the utilitarian vein that efficiency had advised—valueless in their own right but holding immeasurable value for the study and manipulation of the digestive process itself. This was efficiency logic at its purest and foulest: the waste product's essential value lay in its utility as a means to refine digestive processing.

Specifically for Kellogg, the optimal bowel movement product was one measured both in size and frequency—the larger and more often, the better. Three bowel movements a day was a good start; four was closer to optimal. On the pages of *The Stomach*, he described the arrival of these products quite specifically as the necessary signs of the proper processing of the digestive system over the day. On waking up in the morning, he wrote, "the intestinal activity

THE DIGESTIVE TIME TABLE 37

Normal Itinerary of a Meal Passing Through the Alimentary Subway

TIME TABLE

Arrival	Gate	Station	Departure
8:00 A.M.	No. 1. Food Administrator	Mouth	8:30 A.M.
	No. 2. Inspector		
	No. 3. Food and Water		
8:30 A.M.	No. 4. Stomach	Stomach	12:00 Noon
	No. 5. Bowel—Pylorus		
12:00 Noon	No. 6. Ileo Sphincter	Small Intestine	4:00 P.M.
4:00 P.M.	No. 7. Colon—Ileo Valve	Cecum	6:00 P.M.
6:00 P.M.	No. 8. Reversing Gate	Transverse Colon	8:00 P.M.
8:00 P.M.	No. 9. Ejector	Pelvic Colon	10:00 P.M.
	No. 10. Exit	Rectum	10:00 P.M.

SPECIAL NOTICES

Train Late: Held at Stomach Station for 2 hours. Bowel Gate (No. 5) refused to open.
Losing Time: Wreck at Colon Gate (No. 7). Ileocecal valve refuses to close, track obstructed with rubbish. 8 hours late.
Losing Time: Collision with heavy train backing up. 10 hours late.
Losing Time: Obstruction on the track. Ejector Gate (No. 9) refuses to open. 20 hours late.
Losing Time: Serious obstruction. Track buried with rubbish. 35 hours late.
Train arrives at last, after clearing track with dynamite (castor oil), forty hours late.

(This is the usual program when the bowels move only once a day or occasionally.)

FIGURE 1.1. Kellogg's "normal itinerary of a meal passing through the alimentary subway" manifests his obsession with the continuous movement of a meal and the hazards that might slow it down. J. H. Kellogg, *The Itinerary of a Breakfast*, 1919.

naturally set up by the movements of the body" should ensure the remains of yesterday's lunch were well on their way toward the exit. The exciting intestinal actions of breakfast (if on the four-a-day schedule, but lunch, if on the three) likewise would foreshadow the imminent departure/arrival of yesterday's dinner. After dinner, breakfast's itinerary would be completed, having also successfully sped its way through the body's food disassembly line.

Kellogg appended to this wisdom an efficient visual aide: a timetable charting each stop along the "alimentary subway," which showed in quite specific terms the process—now reimagined as a transportation system—that he imagined was taking place in the body's interior (figure 1.1). Food was given a generous twelve to fourteen hours to travel the full length of the line, with the bulk of this time—a good eight hours—devoted to traversing the "nearly twenty-five feet" of intensive processing necessary from mouth to colon. The four to six remaining hours were more than adequate to travel the remaining distance, which was only "one-fifth as great," especially because this final leg required very little processing.[20]

Should food require a full day to travel from the mouth—the digestive system's "entrance gate"—to its exit at the anus, this malfunction would be cause for grave concern and quick repair.[21] For this, Kellogg prescribed "dynamite (castor oil)": the only thing that could "clear the track." (This was "the usual program," he added, "when the bowels move only once a day or occasionally.")[22]

Kellogg's assignment of significance to these bowel movement products did not arrive out of nowhere. His focus on abundance and frequency, and his grave fears of constipation in particular, arose out of a historically specific understanding of the pathological potential of digestion. The rationale for this particular assignment of product, then, and the consequent view of the digestive system as best rationalized and most effectively operating when it was constantly running developed out of Kellogg's dread of bacteria.

The spread of germ theory over the early twentieth century had raised innumerable questions and a great deal of angst about how, where, and why bacteria did their dirty work.[23] As Kellogg ominously described it in his 1918 book *Itinerary of a Breakfast*, when the digestive "train" was held because of a "wreck at the colon gate" or because of a "collision" with another train "backing up" or any number of other food tube disasters the mind could conjure up, the foodstuffs that comprised that train would sit, rotting on the track, just as they would outside the body. This kind of putrefaction was intolerable—the cause of so much harm, both within and outside the food tube. If these bacteria were allowed to linger in the digestive tract, they could then find their way into other parts of the body, producing the systemic crisis that Kellogg referred to as "autointoxication."[24]

In this way, then, just as Fletcher's choice of product—or, rather, absence of product—reflected his own personal understanding of the process he was aiming to rationalize, so too did Kellogg's, which reflected a different set of historically specific anxieties that proliferated in his moment.

Childbirth

Childbirth is in many ways an infinitely thornier example of the process-product nexus in this period, in large part because it already has a clear-cut industrial history attached to it. In this view, childbirth is understood as part and parcel of a problematic rendering of human reproduction in the terms of industrial production.[25] As Barbara Duden influentially explained, the term *reproduction* was coined in the nineteenth century, arising from the movement of production "into the center of political economy." As a way of knowing and describing significance, production remade childbirth in its own image: reimagining its sole purpose as the replication of a labor force and reconceptualizing the potential of the body for birth as merely a sign of the "natural origin of economic concepts."[26] Even now, this narrative exerts substantial political pull so that to dissect the processes that putatively made up this "medicalized childbirth" is to give the appearance of its defense. Likewise, to describe an industrial logic of childbirth is presumed only to rehash a point that Duden and others had settled decades ago.[27]

The tracing of the operative logic of efficiency here does not undo these narratives or the power they hold for understanding the implicit biases of modern medicine. Instead, it demonstrates how this operative logic of medicine also helped to shape a view of childbirth that emphasized the birthing body's experience. That is, many obstetricians explicitly designed their rationalized versions of childbirth *not* with the presumptive product of childbirth—a baby—in mind. Instead, they focused their attention on the health of the birthing body. Though the product-process nexus again indicates the rather arbitrary selection of a product in order to pursue a particular course of process rationalization, the example of childbirth also begins to show a clear preference within medicine to see products as Ford did: not the end point to which processes should be geared but an object that gained its significance precisely insofar as it manifested the qualities of its rationalized process.

Maternal mortality was a clear and well-established problem in the early twentieth century.[28] For some, this problem stemmed from a reading of industry as having tainted birthing bodies to such a degree that they no longer contained the capacity to *do* natural things. This was indeed the view of the obstetrician Grantly Dick-Read, who made this point using a vivid, if highly suspect, comparison between "industrialized" birth and those births that took place in the so-called primitive cultures he had encountered in his travels. In the multiply discriminatory terms of the time, Dick-Read claimed that in these "primitive" societies, birth was naturally easy and painless and largely problem-free.[29] As he described (or imagined) it, natural birth was just one more life event, taking place in between the other "primitive" activities with which the day was filled. One simply squatted briefly so that nature could take its course—a phenomenon that Dick-Read claimed to have witnessed—and then returned to the usual routine, now only with a baby in tow.[30] Industrialization had essentially ruined this process, so affecting the minds of child bearers that they no longer knew how childbirth worked. For the modern woman, Dick-Read explained, "parturition is almost invariably the first primitive, fundamental physical act which she is called upon to perform." It was no wonder, then, that "she" did not know how to do it.[31]

For others, the answer to the problem of childbirth lay in industry itself. As one writer saw it, the problems of childbirth were so similar to those taking place on the assembly line that they too would be solved "by the same methods employed in producing high-grade grain, live stock and manufactured goods."[32] And this was indeed the operative idea behind the work of the prominent obstetrician Joseph B. DeLee, who took on the problem of maternal mortality in the most industrial way possible: by assigning it the position of the product his rationalization of childbirth could uniquely obtain.

DeLee's remaking of childbirth, then, was largely geared toward the production of an ideal healthy mother. Though this view suffuses DeLee's obstetric oeuvre, it was in a widely read and still oft-quoted article in the *American Journal of Obstetrics and Gynecology* in 1920 that he set out the most detailed rationale of the need for such a systemic overhaul. It began with a rather provocative discussion of why childbirth had to be considered a "pathogenic" process—not connected to the health of the babies but rather to the injuries suffered by the mother in childbirth. These were oftentimes so traumatic, he described, that they might be appropriately likened to those acquired by "fall[ing] on a pitchfork and driv[ing] the handle through her perineum."[33] An injury of this magnitude acquired some other way, he explained, would not be viewed as "normal." But they were in birth. He continued:

> Perhaps laceration, prolapse and all the evils are, in fact, natural to labor and therefore normal in the same way as the death of the mother salmon and the death of the male bee in copulation, are natural and normal. If you adopt this view, I have no ground to stand on, but, if you believe that a woman after delivery should be as healthy, as well as anatomically perfect as she was before, and that the child should be undamaged, then you will have to agree with me that labor is pathogenic, because experience has proved such ideal results exceedingly rare.[34]

The failure of the natural processing of birth was thus rendered primarily in terms of its inability to produce its intended products: a woman that was "healthy" and "anatomically perfect," as well as an "undamaged" child. A damaged product called for a processing fix: a rationalizing overhaul of the entire childbirthing system. This is precisely what DeLee provided, in a process he called the "prophylactic forceps operation."

DeLee's procedure of choice remade almost every aspect of the birth process *and* demanded that this process be accomplished, as its title suggested, prophylactically. It was to be deployed *before* the particulars of the birth situation were known or could be ascertained. Indeed, as in the factory, it was out of the question that any system, once rationalized, could allow previous incarnations to make an appearance. Accordingly, as DeLee made clear, there should be no option for some other version of childbirth. Allowing them would be to return to process that, in material terms, produced maternal injury, which, according to his lengthy list, included "perineal tears, prolapsed uteri, recto-vaginal fistulas," as well as eclampsia, postpartum hemorrhage, uterine rupture, puerperal fever, and septicemia.[35]

Much of DeLee's concern with childbirth was its unpredictability. Natural childbirth happened in different ways for different people, leading to endless permutations of complications. DeLee's procedure aimed to obviate even the possibility of any problem by reducing this unpredictability. Rationalizing this process would, the logic went, impose on it a uniformity that would guarantee uniformly perfect products. This is surely why DeLee was so chagrined by the fact that he could not approximate cervical dilation. Indeed, said DeLee, this was the only thing he could not artificially re-create. This fly in the ointment injected a constant level of risk and uncertainty into his procedures, which, in turn, constantly threatened to undo all the uniformity of product his process sought in practice.[36] And it rendered his rationalized process necessarily incomplete.

Despite this, DeLee's procedure was exceedingly popular among those with the financial resources to consume his prophylactic forceps operation, now itself viewed as a process that was a marketable and consumable medical product. He earned himself the patronage of an admiring coterie of wealthy and politically important women, which served him well.[37] Indeed, the prophylactic forceps operation was popular among the middle and upper classes: a fact that should not surprise us, given that these were the women who could afford it. They were also the women that the eugenicists of the period lost the most sleep over. If their modern bodies succumbed to childbirth, the population would become quickly unbalanced by the profusion of children from the working or destitute classes.[38]

One of DeLee's more important patrons was Teddy Roosevelt's scandalous daughter, Alice Roosevelt Longworth, who chose his method of delivery for the birth of her daughter Paulina in 1925. The trendsetter's subsequent endorsement of DeLee's procedure carried no small weight, and it was at her suggestion that the women's magazine *The Delineator* invited DeLee to write two general articles on childbirth in 1926. Featured at the beginning of the first of these, entitled "Before the Baby Comes," was a photo of Longworth holding her "charming Paulina," the visual proof of the political and medical legitimacy of DeLee's methods (figure 1.2).[39] In short time, DeLee's process had vaulted him to the status of a celebrity doctor.

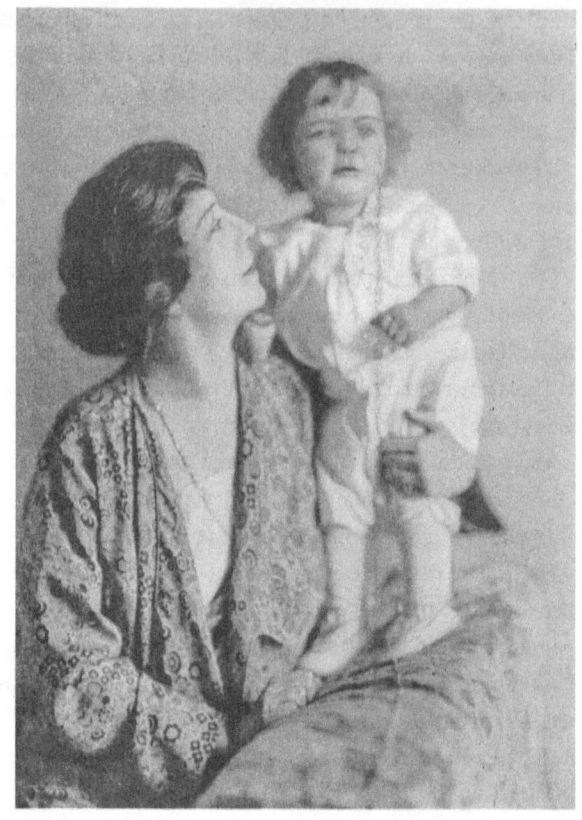

FIGURE 1.2. DeLee's 1926 article "Before the Baby Comes" in the women's magazine *The Delineator* opened with this image of Alice Roosevelt and her "charming little daughter, Paulina." Image courtesy of the Smithsonian Library and Archives, Washington, DC.

Though DeLee is best known probably for his industrial fixes to the problems of wealthy white women, DeLee is also—but complicatedly—hailed as the founder of the Chicago Maternity Center (and before that the Maxwell Street Dispensary), which were free clinics that provided prenatal care and home births for the residents of one of Chicago's poorest and most ethnically diverse neighborhoods. It was this DeLee who was featured by the popular science writer Paul de Kruif in his 1938 book *The Fight for Life* and then again in Pare Lorenz's film of the same name in 1940, made possible by the largesse of Franklin Roosevelt's New Deal government. Heralded here as a saver of mothers, the very same moniker he also received for the work he did to industrialize birth among the wealthy elite he served, DeLee's obstetric work manifested the exclusionary racial logic of efficiency more broadly.

DeLee was a eugenicist in a way that Dick-Read would have approved of. His notion of a two-tiered obstetric care system, where the wealthy white elite gave birth in relative luxurious hospitals while a racially and ethnically diverse array of poor women gave birth at home, captures the divisions of society that efficiency helped to prop up. But it also captures one of the characteristic fixes that efficiency adherents often applied to compensate for efficiency's exclusionist tendencies. Poor and nonwhite women's bodies were not subject to efficiency or industrial logics, so they could not take advantage of the social mobility it offered, nor could they benefit from its egalitarian ethos. But this didn't mean that they were neglected altogether, at least not always. Funded by the donations of the same wealthy elite who enjoyed his industrialized maternity services, DeLee committed himself and his center to provide obstetric care for all. Indeed, his dedication to caring for these women was both personally motivated and deeply felt. But it was also, nonetheless, overtly eugenicist, overtly racist, and ultimately overtly antagonistic to the very values of egalitarianism and democracy that efficiency was thought to hold up.[40]

By the 1930s, the notion that a total remake of childbirth as a process was the right solution to its pathogenic character was well established among its intended and exclusive wealthy white consumers. A 1938 *Reader's Digest* article titled "Our Streamlined Baby" cemented the relationship between birth's remake and its product, maternal health, by celebrating the accomplishment of what Dick-Read had suggested was the ideal of childbirth, its subsuming into the banality of life. Rather than squatting to deliver the baby and returning to work, however, the modern woman would take in a matinee and an early dinner and then check into the hospital for the night. The next morning, she would find the product of her doctor's labor—her baby—at her side.[41]

Despite its popularity among well-to-do women, DeLee's work was not uniformly popular with the obstetrical community. The prevailing logic for obstetrical powerhouses like J. Whitridge Williams of Johns Hopkins was "watchful expectancy," the long-standing principle that those attending births ought only to intervene if necessary. Though in part Williams may have been reflecting an ideological view that childbirth existed outside the industrial logics of the day, his objection also squarely reflected the chaotic nature of obstetrics at the time. Placing too many techniques into the hands of undertrained, inexperienced practitioners who were the far more frequent attendees at childbirths in the United States in this period was simply bad practice. For DeLee's process to supplant natural childbirth and the watchful expectancy principle, the obstetrics community would require a massive upskilling, followed by the thorough and complete dissemination of DeLee's methods.[42]

Williams's concerns, though not necessarily solely addressed to DeLee, certainly found a target in his work. Though DeLee worked energetically to disseminate his procedure, making an enormous set of teaching films between the late 1920s and his death in 1942, it is doubtful that a great many practitioners could have picked it up, both because of the attendant difficulties of learning by film and the sheer complexity of DeLee's procedures.[43] For all of its intent to rationalize and streamline childbirth, DeLee's hallmark prophylactic forceps procedure was exceedingly complicated, requiring the careful administration of at least four drugs at varying times over the course of the procedure as well as an obligatory episiotomy incision, the mastery of implements like forceps and suction catheters, a variety of maneuvers and manual techniques, the existence of acute and learned observational skills, the proper initial care of the baby, the proper inspection of the placenta, and, finally, the careful sewing up of the episiotomy incision, which promised the return to the perfect health—to "virginal conditions," he rather disturbingly specified—that was his trademark guarantee.[44]

Though DeLee's filmic oeuvre did not successfully crack the market on medical distance learning, his films wonderfully manifest the extent to which the rationalization of process took hold in medicine. There are few examples of the outcomes or "products" of the procedures shown on film. On occasion, a smiling new mother appears at the film's end. And in one especially memorable instance, four "cesones," children born by his variant of the cesarean section, are paraded out and lauded as "better physically and mentally" than those "delivered from below" (figure 1.3).[45] But by and large, in these films, it is process that takes center stage: its own qualities and features themselves the guarantor that this was birth done right.

DeLee's fascination with film technology, which saw him at one point touring Hollywood sets "to inspect their big equipment and cross-examine cameramen," highlights its importance to him as a kind of obstetric tool. Film technology was well suited to the task not because it had anything to do with practical obstetrics but because it allowed for the more complete rationalizing of process.[46] DeLee's films required multiple "actors" (DeLee had required, he said, fifteen women to make his cesarean film), high-quality lights and cameras, a cameraperson, scripts, and rehearsals. And when sound came into common use, he added a studio for the creation of sound effects and the recording of voiceovers. The right birth process, it seemed, required not just a flurry of activity in real life but the embrace of a cinematic universe that alone enabled the control over process that could produce DeLee's desired result: a mother's complete return to health. What emerged from DeLee's studio was never, then, the real-time results of what had happened in any given procedure; rather, it was the highly produced, perfectly rationalized process that could *only* be accomplished in a film studio.[47] Filmmaking provided for DeLee the right set of implements with which to perform his rationalization of childbirth, allowing him—through editing—to control even that most recalcitrant of elements, cervical dilation.

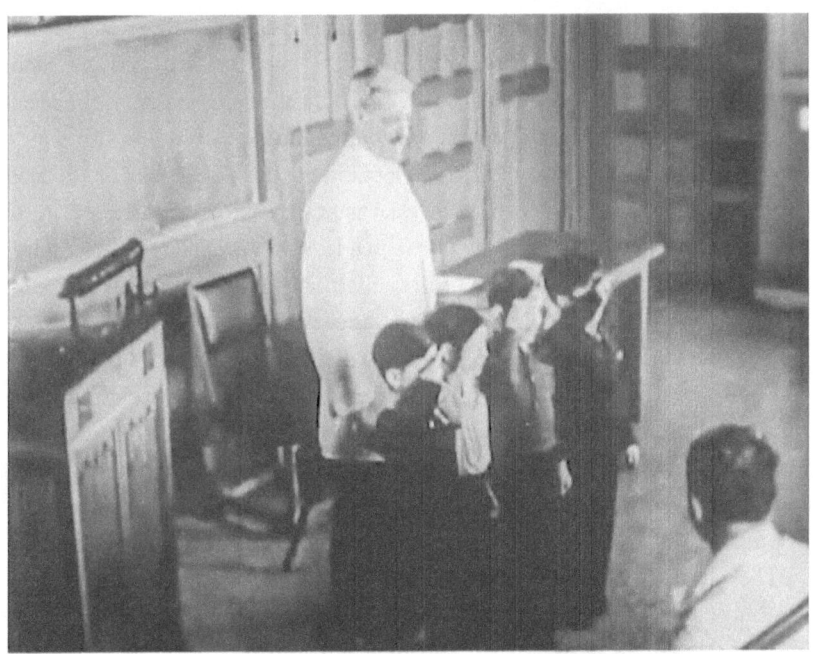

FIGURE 1.3. DeLee's parade of the products of his cesarean section: the "cesones." Film still from Joseph B. DeLee, dir., *Science and Art of Obstetrics: Laparotrachalotomy or Low Cervical Section*, 1936.

The result of these films in real time was not the sea change in obstetric practice that DeLee hoped would come from the dissemination of his techniques. Of course, these filmic techniques also could not achieve any results on their own. Nor did they have any real analogues in day-to-day actual practice. Nonetheless, DeLee persisted, fanatical in his attention to the details of his films, as though to suggest that the only place where complete processing rationalization could exist for childbirth was in the highly edited, highly manipulated world of film and that, perhaps more to the point, the thing that *mattered* most in medicine was the perfection of this processing, whether or not it had any impact whatsoever on the "products" who were supposed to benefit from it.

Process *as* Product: Finale

Just as the body's various processes signaled an obvious opening for the application of industrial rationalization, so too did the overlaps between the factory and the hospital (or, in this case, the clinic) suggest that much could be resolved by paying attention to the product-process relationship.

Indeed, this was just what a 1916 article on outpatient or "dispensary" work in the *Modern Hospital* implied. Though most likely written satirically, the sociologist and health activist Michael M. Davis published this vision of the ideal dispensary as itself a kind of factory without comment (Davis was also director of the Boston Dispensary). This was a place, the article emphasized, where "raw materials"—patients in need of treatment—came to be processed. And though people had to rely on their "personal legs" to enter the building, once inside, these appendages became nearly superfluous. Moving stairways would instead meet the bulk of a patient's conveyance needs.[48]

As patients, the "raw materials" of this health factory ascended up the several floors of the dispensary structure, attended to on the way by a quickly shifting rotation of dispensary personnel: first, a technician to collect and analyze fingerprints for identification purposes; next, a social worker trained to decode their clothing and general bearing in order to ascertain their ability to pay; and finally, a worker who would assign the patient to the relevant clinic.

These escorts would join on one floor and hop off on the floor above, returning to the floor below by a network of poles and chutes that kept the flow of workers moving at pace with their patient raw materials. Patients, meanwhile, would continue their upward journey until they reached the very top of the building, where a clerk would receive them, armed with an updated record (shot ahead of patients using a state-of-the-art pneumatic tube system), and send them on their way down again to visit the clinics as they descended through and out the dispensary's exit. The conspicuous absence of any reference to clinical care placed the article right on trend, presenting processing, not clinical prowess, as the key to medical efficacy.

One commentator who wrote in to express his appreciation of the article felt for sure that this take on the industrially inflected dispensary was meant to be "facetious": a humorous and enjoyable article that, far from describing any real ideal of dispensary practice, was intended to draw greater attention to dispensary study.[49] What this contributor apparently did not know was that Davis's ideal dispensary already had a real-time analogue in the most famous "dispensary" of them all: the Mayo Clinic.

The Mayo Clinic's first building had opened in 1914, two years before Davis included this ode to the modernist dispensary in his article. Given the clinic's reliance on a modernist processing system for its reputation, it might as well have been the article's inspiration.

Run by the illustrious medical brothers Charles and William Mayo, the Mayo Clinic predated its first purpose-built structure. It is generally dated to the 1880s, when "Dr. Charlie and Dr. Will," as they were colloquially known, took over the solo medical practice that their father, William Worall Mayo, had started when he moved his family to the small hamlet of Rochester, Minnesota, twenty years earlier. Before 1914, the Mayo Clinic rented its accommodations, its staff performing all surgical procedures at nearby St. Mary's Hospital.

In some ways, very little changed with the move to the new building. The personnel remained the same, and its reliance on St. Mary's continued. The purpose of this relocation was not, then, to gain space in order to add its own hospital or surgical facilities on-site. Instead, the move to the new building specifically facilitated the diagnostic methods that the Mayos had adopted in their practice. This method was known as the "group practice" or "cooperative" method of diagnosis.[50]

Group practice encapsulated the contemporary emphasis on thorough processing. This was not just a once-over by a single doctor. In the group practice system, patients moved from specialist to specialist, each one offering the testing and examination of a different body part or system until the processing was complete. As one Mayo physician proudly put it:

> Every method known to all the sciences, as they are discovered day by day, is used upon each applicant to determine precisely what ails him or her. No separate or individual part of the sufferer's anatomy escapes the vigilant and thorough search of this commission on diagnosis.[51]

The Mayo Clinic was not the system's only proponent. In fact, the system was sometimes attributed to the prominent physician and "Boston Brahmin" Richard Cabot of the Massachusetts General Hospital. But the system was made most famous at Mayo. Or, perhaps more accurately, the system made the Mayo Clinic famous. Though Dr. Charlie and Dr. Will were beloved in their own right, what made the long and complicated trip to this small and unlikely little town in Minnesota—what made it a "medical Mecca," as one commentator put it—was its promise of this thorough processing.[52] At least this was what the physician John Hornsby concluded, having infiltrated the clinic while researching a story he was writing about its appeal.

The undercover Hornsby went to the Mayo Clinic on the pretext of needing a full physical workup in light of his "strenuous work in connection with the war." What he found was that—yes—everyone loved Dr. Charlie and Dr. Will, who were (and still are) spoken of with reverence and admiration whenever mentioned in or near Rochester. But the reason patients made the pilgrimage to that small town was not because of the personal celebrity of the Mayo brothers; rather, it was because of the growing reputation of the Mayo Clinic as the place to obtain a new and critically important medical product: an accurate diagnosis.

As Hornsby put it, the patients he encountered at the Mayo Clinic had been "passed from family practitioner to specialist, from one specialist to another . . . each one with a dozen or more incomplete or unwritten histories of the great tragedy of illness," yet with no greater knowledge of what was wrong with them than they had when they began that process. The great draw of the Mayo Clinic was that these individuals could finally lay down this exhausting task, thanks to the group practice system. They were, he concluded, incredibly grateful for the peace of mind that this group practice system had finally brought, even, as was not infrequently the case, when therapeutically nothing could be done.[53]

Whatever the veneer of objectivity afforded by Hornsby's purported deep cover as a clinic patient, he was hardly unbiased about the Mayo Clinic. He, like the Mayos and others, belonged to a group of medical reformers who were especially interested in ousting the "solo practitioner," a figure characterized as an old-fashioned nineteenth-century medical holdover who relied on experience and intuition in the making of diagnoses. Just as the rationalized processes of the factory were decimating the livelihood of those who worked with their hands, so too was group practice driving solo practitioners out of the marketplace.

This, it was believed, was a good thing. As Cabot explained, the advantages of group practice over the solo practitioner rested on the fact that no single person could retain all that had come be known about medicine.[54] Charles Mayo echoed the sentiment in a talk on "teamwork," noting that group practice, and the rationalization of medical labor it required, had come about as a result of the "rapid advance of medicine during the last fifty years." He added that even "well-known diseases require experts in various lines, in order that the diagnosis may be proved and complications not overlooked."[55] But when the knowledge was divided up between specialists, who could claim unique and comprehensive knowledge over the new rationalized body conceived now as divided into corresponding specialty parts, and when these specialists with their unique knowledge were brought back together, full coverage could once again be achieved.

In some sense, the product of this system was thus an invention of the rationalized process itself. That is, *accurate* diagnosis was not necessarily an obvious candidate for a medical product, since in most cases it promised nothing at all except for a rather circular validation of the rightness of the processing system. Accurate diagnosis was in some sense an invention of group practice, even as it was also used to verify the validity of the group practice process.

The group practice logic thus formed a closed system. There was little outside verification that this process was actually the right one, and no guarantee, aside from the system itself, that the diagnosis reached was actually accurate. Sometimes, but by no means always, the reduction or removal of symptoms would act as verification that the illness had been accurately diagnosed. But for those for whom this accurate diagnosis was a death sentence, as in some of the cases Hornsby described, or for those who learned when receiving their diagnosis that there was no treatment, the acceptance of the accuracy of their diagnosis rested on the patient's willingness to accept that this final product was a desirable one.

Since the system's legitimacy rested on the validity and visibility of its rationalized, complete process, it also makes sense that the new Mayo building would set the group practice system in material, architectural terms.[56] Though its design was made to facilitate patient processing for its own sake, it also made visible to patients the full, rationalized processing that they were, as raw materials, undergoing.

Though the design for the Mayo Clinic's new home was officially attributed to the Minnesota firm Ellerbe & Round, it owed much to Henry S. Plummer, a medical practitioner and Mayo cofounder with a penchant for system design.[57] Plummer's medical strengths were organizational, and he drafted into his hospital blueprints the group practice ethos: that effective medicine and accurate diagnoses were desirable precisely because they were the result and verification of efficient, rationalized processing. Tellingly, Plummer was later celebrated as having so orchestrated the building that he ultimately had designed into existence precisely this new method of practicing medicine that was the group practice system.

That this was the very point of the new clinic building is made clear by the details of its construction. To facilitate the flow of patients through its space, Plummer implemented a series of signal lights, telegraph tickers, and time clocks to control and direct the flow of what Davis's column had referred to as the clinic-factory's "raw materials," the patients.[58] Even air obeyed the metronome as it was sucked inside by the ventilation system, heated or cooled by the fountain in the lobby, sent throughout the building, and recycled every three minutes.[59] Though the initial Mayo building lacked the pneumatic tube system imagined in the ideal dispensary, Plummer's subsequent design, for the second clinic building built fourteen years later, corrected this error. Pneumatic tubes plus a proprietary telephone system ensured that information now moved as quickly and efficiently as the patients.

Indeed, Plummer's engineering prowess quite effectively manifested the processing ethos of group practice. This was a fact that the sixteen hundred guests who gathered on the clinic's opening day learned when they were whisked away for a tour that led them down the clinic's processing route that they might follow one day themselves.

As they navigated through this structured environment, visitors experienced its precise choreography of ascending and descending—right stairwells

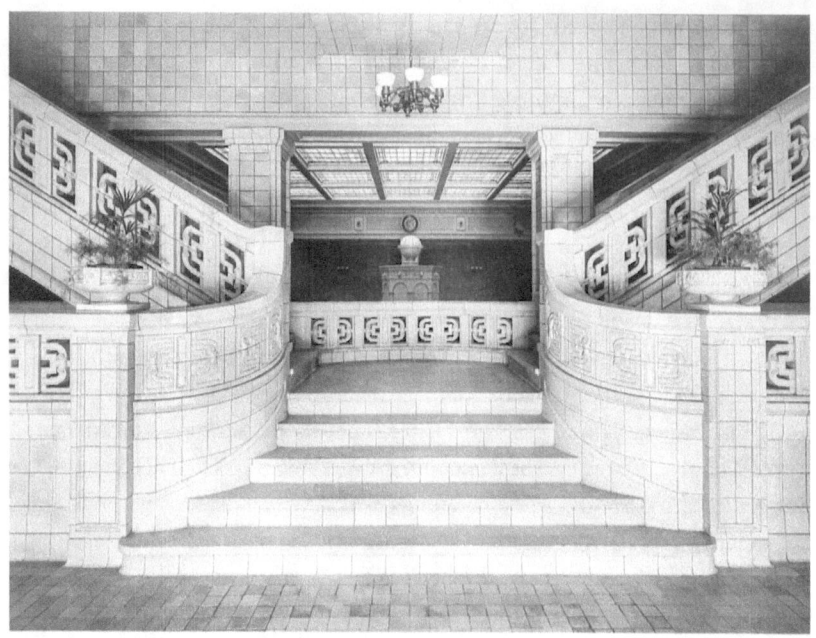

FIGURE 1.4. The grand central staircase of the Mayo Clinic Building, ca. 1914. Image courtesy of the Mayo Historical Unit, Mayo Clinic, Rochester, Minnesota.

were for going up, left for down, ensuring that those arriving did not mix with those leaving and everyone was always turning to the left (figure 1.4). Though the slides and poles that dropped staff back down from floor to floor in Davis's imagined dispensary proved a bridge too far for the clinic, the circulatory motion of physicians was ensured by the call lights that lit up to bring a wanted physician to a particular examination room. Each physician had an assigned color, and each set of colored lights appeared in each room. It was a simple matter, then, of pressing one of these buttons, which not only lit up the light over the door but activated the lights throughout the structure, guiding the wanted physician to the proper floor and then, through a series of hall lights, to the proper room. While patients moved in only one direction, physicians attentively circulated around them, all with the same goal in mind: to produce of these raw materials the promised finished products.[60]

Newspaper accounts also focused their attention on the building's processing propensity, lauding the new clinic building as "the acme of perfection" and the "culmination of the highest ideals" of medicine in part for its great "systematicity."[61] And though these accounts included attention to the high-tech additions to the Mayo Clinic building—the state of the art X-ray department, for example—the tendency of these reports was to trace the tour route that those who had been lucky enough to attend in person had also followed. Here, as elsewhere, the processing ethos of the clinic held primacy of place.

Against the backdrop of the current Mayo Clinic—or, really, any hospital or outpatient setting—it may be difficult to imagine this early twentieth-century logic of rationalized processing as the guarantor of diagnostic accuracy or therapeutic success. Indeed, especially given our contemporary attachment to the notion that effective care is "patient-centered," the notion that patients would flock to the Mayo Clinic precisely for its impersonal über-systematized experience feels foreign to our sensibilities now. Yet, it was processing power, not clinical genius, that made the Mayo Clinic such a paragon of effectiveness, reportedly earning it over $1 million annually in the years after the building opened.[62]

In light of the fuller picture of the significance of processing for health in the period, the group practice system makes sense. Given the ubiquity of process rationalization as a solution to the thorny problems both of industry and work and, as outlined here, of digestion and childbirth, it is not surprising that the group practice diagnostic system would emerge, as these others also had, as the right solution. Physicians in the early twentieth century thus looked to process to solve the problem of medical effectiveness, implicitly establishing it as the "product of medicine" that, as Gilbreth and Codman had noted, was required if medicine was to be truly modern.

2

The Factory

The Ford Hospital? Sure, I know all about it. They put you through there, all right. You just get undressed and sit down on a moving belt, just like you was a flivver. The doctors line up along the belt, and as you go through each guy does his bit. It ain't like the old way when one doctor did everything. At the end of the belt you're through, and they slide you right onto a bed that's got a little flivver engine and it takes you right away to your room. Great, ain't it?—A (POSSIBLY APOCRYPHAL) DETROIT BELLBOY IN 1924, quoted in Crowther, "The Real Story of Ford's Hospital"

Since 1903, when the Ford Motor Company opened its doors in Detroit, Michigan, its products have occupied a special place in American culture. Gertrude Stein liked to write in the passenger seat of a Model T that she called "Auntie." The Model A was the vehicle of choice for running moonshine during Prohibition. Dr. Martin Luther King Jr. drove a Ford-made Lincoln, President John Kennedy was assassinated in one, and President Ronald Reagan was shot outside of one. In *Bullitt*, Steve McQueen drove a Mustang like a man possessed, and in

Thelma and Louise, Susan Sarandon and Geena Davis drove their Thunderbird off the edge of the Grand Canyon. The Beach Boys' "Little Deuce Coupe" was a Ford Model 18.

More complicated is the figure of Henry Ford himself. As the founder of one of the most successful American companies of all time, he occupies a sanctified place in the annals of American business history. In other parts of culture, his status is less certain. A notorious anti-Semite and union-buster, he looms invisible but large in *Brave New World* as the progenitor of its dystopia, holds the singular honor of being the only American to be favorably name-dropped in *Mein Kampf*, and is condemned for his efforts against unions in Upton Sinclair's *The Flivver King*. His own literary legacy includes a tract about the dangers of smoking called *The Case against the Little White Slaver*, a memoir, and a collection of serialized racist conspiracy theories called *The International Jew*. In the 1960s, the US Postal Service included Henry Ford in its Prominent Americans commemorative stamp series.

And then there are Ford's pioneering principles and methods of mass production, collectively termed "Fordism." In the context of both business and labor history, Fordism looms larger than Ford, although its significance is differently inflected in each. In both histories, however, Fordism is placed squarely in the lineage of Taylorism—the management techniques of Ford's early contemporary Frederick Winslow Taylor. Together, the two systems are often viewed as key and only trivially different exemplars of American industrial capitalism of the early twentieth century, remaking the world of work into one where routinization and surveillance became the rule and giving rise to the society and economy of mass consumption that we continue to inhabit.[1]

The seeming intrinsic paradoxes of Fordism abound. Ford introduced the $5 day and the five-day workweek, giving workers at Ford's plant far better pay and more leisure time than were available elsewhere. At the same time, the company deployed a racist and xenophobic "sociological department" that enforced the requirement that workers who received these benefits were married, eschewed both alcohol and tobacco, and followed exacting standards of cleanliness (as determined by unannounced home visits).[2] It was an approach that early twentieth-century social theorist Antonio Gramsci saw not only as an essential part of Ford's own success, but also as the new, dominating form of capitalism emanating from the United States.[3] According to Gramsci, as well as those scholars revisiting Gramsci's interpretation in the 1970s, the principles and techniques of Fordism were the story of American capitalism writ large. Predicated on exercising control over the working class that was as absolute as it was restrictive, this system could not grow without the "voluntary submission" of workers to its "labor discipline."[4]

There are Fords, Ford himself and Fordism, and then there is the Henry Ford Hospital, a Ford product that features rarely in the American consciousness or indeed anywhere else. Opened in 1921, its story stands as a confounding companion to Ford's other consumer offerings, not to mention his social ideals and industrial principles. Of course, at a time when Andrew Carnegie and John D. Rockefeller were showering philanthropy on libraries, schools, and other public goods, it seems sensible that an industrial magnate with a keen interest in social transformation, albeit on his own terms, might find a proper avenue for some of his profits in the maintenance of the public's health. But Ford insisted again and again that his hospital was absolutely not a philanthropic endeavor and that, owing to his disdain for the goals of organized philanthropy, he himself was *not* a philanthropist.[5] Rather, he considered the Henry Ford Hospital to be a fully Fordist enterprise—an extension into health care of the principles that undergirded his automobile factory.

In some ways, the Ford Hospital appeared to be quite Fordist, indeed.[6] It was designed by Albert Khan, the same industrial architect responsible for Ford's factories, and it incorporated the latest and greatest of medicine's efficiency technologies, leading to the inevitable comparison of its patients to "flivvers," the contemporary slang term for the Model T.[7] But in its physical design and efficiency infrastructure, the hospital was bog-standard—hardly different from other hospitals of the period on which, in many important ways, it was modeled. Indeed, the logic of industrial efficiency had already pervaded medicine by this time, to the point that a hospital built according to factory efficiency principles—a machine unto itself—was not uniquely Fordist.[8]

If not as a paean to the Fordist philosophy nor a manifestation of Ford's true philanthropic leanings, what should we make of the Henry Ford Hospital? Though a slightly artificial question, it helpfully points to the problem of narrating the overlaps between industrial logics and technologies (here, the factory) and medical knowledge-making practices and institutional setups (here, the hospital) that appear variously throughout the book.

Certainly, taking a fresh look at the Ford Hospital allows us to see where the scholarship on industrial culture has been too reductive. As Stefan Link in his *Forging Global Fordism* has so eloquently pointed out, Fordism as it came to be understood and disseminated was not nearly so "Fordist" in Ford's own hands as it was in Gramsci's. That is, Ford's own philosophy, particularly visible in the first two decades of the twentieth century, was far more populist: as Link puts it, it was a movement both "at odds with the emphasis on extraction and producer goods that characterized America's Second Industrial Revolution" and "subversive of the economic hierarchies that found their expression in the grand alliance of finance and industrial capital" that guided the likes of Carnegie and Rockefeller.[9] There is perhaps no greater illustration of the complexity of the Fordist philosophy, at least as it stood in the first couple of decades of the twentieth century, than the Henry Ford Hospital. Neither Fordist in the pejorative sense nor philanthropic in the Rockefellerian sense, the Henry Ford Hospital encapsulated a subversive Fordist worldview that enabled a vision of mass production as a populist, and in this case a therapeutic, entity.

By the same token, this revisitation of the Ford Hospital allows for a new narrative of how medicine was developing over the same period. If the Ford Hospital was an example of populism as a function *of* mass production rather than what Jeanne Kisacky has described as the meeting of industrial capitalism's "technological and economic prowess" with an "egalitarian aspiration" of rather less clear origin, then it makes sense that it should be viewed less as an outlier and more as an instructive manifestation of what was *already* populist about those medical-factory overlaps inspired by medical efficiency proponents and already prominent in the mainstream of medicine of this era.[10]

This folding together of medicine and industry, with its emphasis on mass production as a vehicle for populism, suggests that, at least to some degree, industrial efficiency helped introduce into medicine a vision of what good care ought to look like, rather than serving as care's antithesis. It highlights the surprising flexibility and experimental quality of this period's enthusiasm for efficiency, adding to the story of medicine's industrialization a kind of egalitarianism—or at least a populism—that contributed to the vision of what medicine was and could be. It is a story that jockeys for position with the story told more commonly about medicine in this period, as one moving increasingly toward professionalization and the cementing and distancing of medical expertise from a general public.

The Henry Ford Hospital

Though the number of sources that describe the Ford Hospital in detail are few, the general schema of the hospital is well known. This is largely because it is by most accounts not an especially unique example, even if its connections to Ford seem to make it an enticing example of industrial influence in medicine. That is, the Ford Hospital does not hold a special place in the modernist tradition of hospitals of this period, at least as far as design goes. As most accounts make clear, the institution followed the well-established path of medical modernity already trodden by the best hospitals of its era, including the Mayo Clinic (curiously also under-described in comparison with its relative importance), the Johns Hopkins

Hospital, the Massachusetts General Hospital, and many others both large and small that were reorganized, revamped, or rebuilt over this period.

What we know specifically about the Henry Ford Hospital is generally told in terms of how it became Ford's project, since its acquisition was out of keeping with the usual interests of the industrialist. And though this reading is quite often folded into a view of Ford the philanthropist—for his outlying concern with such an explicitly nonindustrial enterprise—it is in fact a better fit with the more holistic vision of social welfare through mass production that was characteristic of Ford's other ventures.

Most accounts dwell on the fact that Ford had never expected to own or operate a hospital. As he described it in 1914 to Charles and William Mayo—the famous brothers who ran their own eponymous clinic in Rochester, Minnesota—the fact that he was associated with such a project at all was simply because circumstances had dropped a "hospital in [his] lap."[11] It had all started in 1909, when his personal surgeon William Metcalf, in whom Ford reportedly placed great confidence, solicited his famous patient for a donation to the building fund of the Detroit General Hospital. Metcalf believed that there was a growing need to serve the city's swelling population, which Ford's industrial successes had partly precipitated, especially after his decision to nearly triple wages in 1914. Ford's famous "$5 day" wage had been introduced in January of that year, but even before then, the precipitous growth of the Ford company's operation attracted far more new residents to the city than his factories directly employed.[12]

Population growth was not the only problem on Metcalf's mind. He was also inspired by the growing demand within the medical community to put the proprietary medical schools and what the American Medical Association (AMA) pejoratively referred to as the "irregular institutions" in which graduates of these schools practiced out of business. This was a move that the AMA had been advocating since the turn of the century. As early as 1904, then, Metcalf was promoting the construction of a Detroit hospital that would employ only AMA-approved, and therefore reputable, medical practitioners, presumably those who had *not* been trained at Detroit's two for-profit medical schools. Further, this hospital would not allow "fee-splitters," those who took part in the common practice of collecting kickbacks on referral to medical and surgical colleagues.

By 1912, the hospital project had run into funding problems. Though Ford's own personal confidence in Metcalf led to the industrialist's purchase of the land for the hospital and an additional $10,000 contribution, funds raised elsewhere to support the project failed to match its ambition of a 1,000-bed complex. By 1914, construction had stalled, and the proposed citadel of health stood as an ugly, unfinished blight on Detroit's urban landscape. The first proposed plan to save the project would have seen it merge with one of the proprietary institutions, the Harper Hospital—one of the hospitals to which Metcalf had presented his own as an antidote. The next would have seen the hospital turned over to the city of Detroit to do with what it pleased.

In any event, Ford refused to contribute any further funds to the project. By some accounts, he had broken with Metcalf over some perceived personal wrong. Others suggest he was simply disgusted with the poor management of the hospital project. Further contributions would, after all, have made him the primary benefactor of a project over which he was to have limited, and ever receding, control.

The situation changed in 1914, when Ford abruptly became the outright owner of the new institution. It was an about-face that at least one account traces to a story that appeared in the *Detroit News*, planted by the chair of the hospital committee (and publisher of that paper). The article purportedly painted an unattractive portrait of Ford, ultimately laying the blame for the project's failure at his feet. The purpose had apparently been to shame Ford for his lack of cooperation as a member of the hospital committee.[13]

Reading of himself as a financial failure spurred Ford to action. He sent a letter to the committee on June 2, 1914, requesting that the hospital be turned over to him entirely to run as he saw fit. Ford repaid the other contributors to the project and acquired for himself what would become, by many of these laudatory accounts, Ford's crowning philanthropic achievement (deemed "philanthropic" in large part because it was such an endless financial drain on the otherwise lucrative Ford enterprises): the Henry Ford Hospital.[14]

Ford's initial plans for his new medical institution suggest his lack of interest in the kind of clinical medicine practiced in hospitals of the time. Indeed, when a journalist pressed Ford about his announced plans for building a medical center just a few miles down the road from his first automobile factory, Ford waved off the question, saying that medicine was "'not a bit good for anything.'" He had something very different in mind. "'I am working now,' the industrialist told the reporter, 'to have the doctors in my hospital at Detroit do away with its use altogether.'"[15] Ford was channeling one popular view of medicine at the time—namely, that the very best use of a hospital was to contribute to its own obsolescence.

Giving an example of what this meant in practice, Ford clarified to a different journalist that his hospital would not be the "repair shop . . . to cure disease and care for the wrecks" that most hospitals were. That did nothing to stop disease or prevent bodies from becoming wrecked in the first place. Instead, Ford explained, he was focused on producing very particularly defined "cures": in this particular instance, a cure for cancer. And by cure, he did not mean therapy or treatment after the fact but rather prevention: the Ford Hospital was to prevent disease from ever occurring in the first place by somehow spreading principles of proper diet and discipline, replacing the "intemperance not only of drinking but of eating and thinking" that was, in Ford's mind, cancer's cause.[16]

This focus on prevention brought together Ford's own ideas of health, his understanding of engineering, and the efficiency logic that many at the time considered medicine's best path to efficacy. Indeed, though surgical services had a place in Ford's understanding of medical practice, he placed the highest value on the proper maintenance of the body as an efficient engine. The industrialist famously abstained from alcohol and tobacco, as he also insisted his workers do, and generally preferred, as one of the hospital's physicians recalled, to treat any onset of ill health with therapies such as a "fast ride with a little jouncing around" in the back seat of one of his cars. He also had the unwelcome tendency to warn friends laid up in his hospital against following the advice of its physicians. His quite serious counsel to those suffering from heart disease: "lie on the floor for half an hour twice a day" and "eat celery and carrots."[17]

As part of his efficient lifestyle, Ford was, like many of his contemporaries, a devotee of the school of thought best exemplified by John Harvey Kellogg and Horace Fletcher: namely, that digestion was the bodily process most vital to health. For a while, visitors to Ford's home in Dearborn, Michigan, were treated to various unappetizing lunches, most notably the grass sandwich, which he believed offered a particularly strong laxative effect. Ford experimented with other unusual edibles, believing for a time that another link in the chain of medicine's obsolescence would be the discovery of the "perfect food." Indeed, a critical piece of Ford's plan to cure cancer was his vision for a dietetic department focused on discovering this dietary Shangri-la. This was to be the jewel in the crown of his new hospital.[18]

Ford's concerted interest in the hospital and the cures it might produce was quite often expressed in tandem with his vehement denial that the hospital represented any sort of philanthropic opportunity. In an avowal that doubled as a tacit put-down of the activities of the East Coast industrial capitalists he worked hard to distance himself from, he repeatedly told reporters that he had *not* acquired the hospital merely as a way to "square [himself] with justice by giving money to hospitals" after taking "millions of profit from the work of [his] employees."[19] Instead, the Ford Hospital was going to be a "producer" (of cancer cures through prevention and of other ailments through the invention of the perfect food) just as his factories were.

This goal for the hospital helped to reposition it, not as an institution that Ford sponsored in the same way that Carnegie had purchased libraries or funded colleges, but as a space that had a role to play as part of the larger Fordist philosophy that drove Ford's company more generally. Indeed, Ford further insisted that his hospital would not contain "experts" drawn from clinical medicine, since they would already be tainted in the same kind of way that other businesses were tainted by the burden of business as usual. Instead, the cure to cancer would be invented on the hospital's "shop floor" just as his assembly line had been. As he put it, "'We expect to produce our own experts. We shall begin at the bottom and work with the plant until we educate ourselves and our own force of hospital men as we educated ourselves in the automobile shop.'"[20] In this sense, the hospital was to be a populist institution: one where real ingenuity—as at the heart of efficiency—was crowd-sourced.

While the Ford Hospital would mimic its industrial counterpart in its productive methods, in Ford's early imaginings it had another, more discrete role to play as part of the larger Ford organization. Ford's comments about cancer came at the same time that John Lee, the director of the Ford Sociological Department, claimed that another reason for Ford's acquisition was to extend the work of what newspapers sometimes called his "welfare department." In short, the project was tethered to the larger and more holistic, albeit systematically insidious, social program that the Ford Motor Company subjected its workers to.

The Ford Sociological Department is well known in the literature for its uncomfortable overlapping of care with invasive social control. To be sure, Ford was not alone in this notion of "welfare work," as it was called by the National Civic Organization. The importance of these types of programs was built into the progressivist rhetoric of the time, which argued for the improvement of workers' lives by the addition of services extended beyond the confines of the workday.[21] To Ford, the introduction of the $5 day wage carried the opportunity to shape the lives and habits of workers to fit the requirements for receiving the wage, paired with a responsibility to help those who would not know what to do with such a sudden influx of cash. Of course, the resulting disciplinary practices were heavy-handed, agency-sapping exemplars of the nativist and eugenicist underpinnings of the "Social Gospel."[22]

Indeed, as both Beth Tompkins Bates and Elizabeth Esch have noted, Ford's commitment to hiring Black workers made explicit the sharp edge of his welfare-*cum*-industrial capitalism.[23] Ford was indeed singular in his willingness to hire Black workers and even more singular in his commitment to paying them on par with his white workers. While in some senses a progressive action that integrated Ford's Michigan factories far earlier than any other American automaker, Ford's hiring of Black workers was rooted firmly in what Luther Adams has called his position as a "modern architect of racial capitalism."[24] By hiring Black workers, who, among other things, were routinely excluded from the major autoworker unions and thus would not strike, Ford was able to make the segregationist, racist mores of the day play to his favor.

This same double-edged sword of Fordist efficiency extended to health concerns. One early example was Ford's decision to create a "ward for consumptives" out of a space better known as his car factory's steel tempering room. This was a fifteen-foot space where annealing furnaces produced the hot steel that was subsequently laid to cool on the room's iron floor. Realizing that it had a "temperature [as] high and the air as dry as in the desert country" to which tuberculosis patients were routinely sent, Ford felt he had discovered a marvelously efficient use of space and energy. He could place tubercular patients in among the hot steel and hotter furnaces, allowing workers the full experience of a therapeutic climate, he said, while also preventing them from doing what he imagined went on in a sanatorium: a lot of thumb-twiddling and illness bemoaning. In a mindset where productivity and happiness were closely allied, this "industrial sanatorium" seemed a perfect solution.[25]

But one needn't be a cynic to see that it was also clearly a way to keep workers working, possibly at the expense of the time they needed to heal, and certainly at the expense of any sort of choice about where and how to heal. At a moment when worker retention posed a constant problem, reimagining the hot, dry, therapeutic air of Arizona as a by-product of a key work process at the Ford Factory was a classically Fordist solution in the most pejorative sense: a problematically controlling intervention that stripped workers of their right to therapies—even illness experiences—that sat outside the Fordist universe.

This consistently uncomfortable combination of care and control permeated the work of the Ford Sociological Department, which had been set up in tandem with the $5 day wage. Implemented in part to solve the problem of high labor turnover in the factory after the introduction of Ford's production line, the wage increase was accompanied by the division of the working day into three shifts of eight hours each. The factory could thus run twenty-four hours a day while each worker would be paid $5 for one shift a day, six days a week.[26] Ford was clear that this wage, which was far higher than the wages paid at other, similar factories, was not charitable. Though it has been (and was at the time) widely described instead as a form of profit-sharing, Ford was inconstant also in this description. In 1915, he told business entrepreneur Roger Babson that the $5 day wage was more about social justice than it was about the sharing of profits per se. "I don't understand why the newspapers and magazines insist upon referring to our 'profit sharing plan,'" Ford carped to Babson, since that would require "a division of the profits in accordance with the respective efforts or producing qualities of the different department and men in them . . . founded in statistics and records designed to show to whom the profits are due."²⁷

The $5 day wage was to be something different: a higher wage derived from profits but based on the much simpler accounting that the Ford assembly-line worker, like any worker, ought to receive enough money from his work to support his family and live comfortably. If wages were "largely a matter of custom," as Ford declared them to be, then his was an effort to change the custom—to pay a living wage to all (who met the requirements) because that would drive the economy more readily than would charity or, really, any true profit-sharing arrangement. The point was to create a stable class structure where charity was unnecessary and where the square deal reigned.²⁸ This was a move, then, that was—at least as Ford styled it sometimes—fundamentally about socioeconomic leveling.²⁹

Ford had famously stringent requirements to be met to qualify for his $5 day wage, which, as one journalist put it, chiefly boiled down to living by the "gospel of cleanliness and thrift."³⁰ To ensure that Ford workers met this standard, the sociological department's "65 investigators in 65 cars with 65 drivers" (though in other publications this number was variously described) were sent out each day to investigate the roughly 30 percent of Ford employees who had applied for the wage but had not been accepted in the first six months.³¹ Those in this group had six months to get their lives together and meet the Ford employee standard or they would be fired.³² Attending also to this group was a legal department and a fleet of physicians who followed up each day with those who did not show up to work. The role of these investigators was purportedly not punitive: they were tasked with assessing and then repairing the family lives of workers so that they could reach their full productive potential and thus be included in the $5 day wage.³³

Though both secondary and even some contemporary accounts have pointed to the problematic nature of these Ford company welfare policies, not least their underlying nativism, the public stories that described the activities of the welfare department—thanks in large part to savvy marketing on the part of the Ford company—pressed on the themes of transformation and uplift.³⁴ There was nary a story in the papers that did not end with a clean, healthy, and happy Ford worker in a happy and healthy new home, typically accompanied by a happy and healthy wife and a set of smiling, carefree children.

It was in this vein that Ford thought his hospital could function within the Fordist cosmos, at least initially. The hospital would serve the same community from which he drew both his workers and consumers (with the $5 day wage and his sociological department, workers would also become good consumers) through a blending of what Link has described as the welfare capitalism of the nineteenth century with the industrial capitalism of the twentieth century. It was a logic that embodied the conflicted goals of efficiency more broadly.[35]

The Hospital Factory

Ford's initial vision of a hospital that would focus on the prevention of, or cures for, disease while rescuing bodies from moral and physical inefficiency did not come to fruition. When the hospital did fully open in December of 1921, after briefly being used to treat war casualties during World War I and later aiding the city of Detroit during the final wave of the Spanish flu pandemic in 1920, it operated as a more conventional hospital. Perhaps as a result, he ultimately put the day-to-day clinical operations into the hands of his personal secretary, Ernest Liebold.

Where Ford did retain at least some control, however, was in the development of the hospital's physical and administrative footprint. At least this was how Ford's contributions were billed in the papers. Though there was one key element of the Ford Hospital that was suffused with the Fordist philosophy, there were few, if any, discernible design or bureaucratic elements that were actually *new* in the Ford Hospital. Of course, this did not stop both Ford's supporters and critics from finding signs everywhere of Ford's influence.

Of the original plans, only the first, already partially built structure at the site was completed. The remainder of the hospital plant and the planned new building were designed by the industrial designer Albert Khan, who had also designed Ford's factories. Although this detail alone might distinguish the Ford Hospital from others of the same period—and certainly journalists made much hay of the fact that a factory planner had designed a hospital—the new premises were more an exemplar of contemporary thinking in modern hospital design than they were an industrial outlier. At the time and in retrospect, the pneumatic tubes, pipes, ducts, tunnels, and other time-saving devices installed in the Ford Hospital that gave it the appearance of being fully industrial (and, perhaps ominously, even Fordist) were already and ostentatiously on display in the most celebrated of American medical institutions.[36] Indeed, the pages of medical management journals described such technologies as an expected and necessary part of modern best practices.[37]

Some journalists were attuned to this reality and ably traced the supposed Fordist lineages of the hospital back to other major medical institutions that were its precedent. But for others, the very fact that Ford had opened a hospital was enough to launch a discourse around the dangers of applying industry to medicine. The assembly-line rhetoric was simply irresistible: critics variously warned that the Ford Hospital would treat the sick like Model Ts or flivvers, with patients literally placed on a moving production line and moved mechanically and heartlessly through what was really a factory disguised as a house of healing.

Ford's supporters also made much of his purported involvement in a hospital, touting its elements of modernity to those who were already inclined to favor Ford's methods. One feature that got quite a lot of press was the Ford Hospital's decision to create uniform private rooms. As newspapers tended to report it, Ford had been dismayed by the lack of routine and order at the Detroit General Hospital building that he had inherited, most upsettingly manifested in the idiosyncratic mix of "various sized rooms" and small wards it contained. Rather than return to the architects who had assembled this inefficient monstrosity, he purportedly dispatched engineers from the factory to guide the plans for the new building.[38]

Most accounts insist that Ford was uniquely responsible for this redesign and that his industrial mindset played a key part of the decision-making. In one common anecdote, Ford asked the physicians recruited to work at his hospital what they considered the "fundamental unit" of a hospital to be. After much hemming and hawing, they were said to have replied that they "supposed . . . it was the patient's room." With the view that "the whole plan for building a hospital should be . . . a quantity production of that unit," Ford thus focused his attention on perfecting this single unit so that, in its replication, it would produce the perfect institution.[39]

Dismissive of his physicians' offers to reconstruct the room based on a study of what other prominent hospitals had done, Ford determined to arrive at this perfect unit in a process ripped straight from the factory floor, the site from which the tenets of mass production had emerged and were constantly being upgraded by a system of trial and error. He would give "the men who had been selected to head the staffs a carpenter and some wall board" so that they could "work out an ideal hospital room and bath—a room which would have all the space needed and none over."[40] They should invent this room themselves, in other words, by mocking up different prototypes, exactly as Ford's engineers had done on the shop floor to arrive at his Model T's final version.

After a series of variously configured rooms had been built, he and his design staff decided on a room measuring 16' × 10' (or, more precisely, 9'10") with its own private bath. This became the base unit for the hospital, which ultimately comprised about 600 identical private rooms.[41] As many have observed, the result was a hospital that, like the Ford Factory, was intentionally "replicative and regular, with a symmetry and a pervading focus on utility."[42]

Much of this rhetoric appears to have been written either to cultivate publicity for the Ford Hospital or to celebrate Ford himself, insisting as it does on Ford's personal role in designing the hospital, perhaps as a selling point for those who also appreciated his Model T. But redesigning the private patient room was not peculiar to the Ford Hospital. Many others on the vanguard of modern hospital design had already concluded—though the decision was not without contention—that private rooms were both efficient and (therefore) modern and thus belonged in the modern hospital.[43] Many other hospitals already had private pavilions with rooms that were generally uniform in size. Indeed, for all of Ford's emphasis on having invented the ideal room through his mockups, the standard Ford Hospital room was only a couple of inches narrower than the 16′ × 10′1″ standard private rooms at Johns Hopkins.[44] In this respect at least, Ford had done little more than perform a quite showy reinvention of the wheel.

It was ostensibly Ford and not his critics or backers who insisted that the rather more populist efficiency methodology of trial and error used to determine room sizes was distinctively his own. This was indeed the same thought process that had made him promise, before the hospital was built, that his hospital would invent its cures on the hospital "factory floor" rather than bringing in established experts from other hospitals. But in fact here, too, Ford was not inventing but merely implementing the larger, longer traditions of a critical efficiency methodology. The notion of a trial-and-error process as essential to medical efficiency was at the core of the message the industrial efficiency expert Frank Gilbreth delivered to medicine in the early 1910s.[45] It was manifested in the debates about hospital appliances throughout the period, where each new invention vied to become the standard that other appliances would then seek to improve on.[46] But its clearest manifestation was almost certainly to be found in the work of the American College of Surgeons, whose hospital standardization program rested on this selfsame logic, scaling it up to a national and then briefly international level.

The Johns Hopkins Hospital was likely also the inspiration for the Ford Hospital closed staff—a staff who would practice nowhere other than the Ford—rather than stemming, as Ford told it, from his own personal observation that he would never "ask every person who wants to build a car to come into my factory to build it."[47] The fact that nearly all, if not all, of the Ford Hospital's initial roster of physicians and surgeons had been drawn from Johns Hopkins is suggestive indeed that the Ford Hospital was probably more indebted to its medical predecessors, and to Johns Hopkins in particular, than it was to the Ford plant.[48]

Another key feature that attracted a great deal of attention at the Ford Hospital was its diagnostic unit. Following some of the most prominent medical thinkers of the day—especially the influential Mayo Clinic—the Ford diagnostic unit followed the group practice model, in which a coterie of specialists served on a veritable assembly line of patient treatment, offering test after test until a patient's entire body had been thoroughly examined.[49] Only at that point, once these "raw materials" had made their way through the physician assembly line, could a diagnosis be made.[50] The evidence that a diagnosis was accurate was to be found, of course, in the thoroughness of the rationalized examination the patient had experienced.

Though the Ford Hospital had adopted the group practice system because of its primacy as a methodology at the country's most important hospitals, it became an important rhetorical landing point for the Detroit medical societies, which decried the group practice method as assembly-line medicine and depicted it as a Fordist intrusion into medicine. The Ford Hospital was a place, they sneered, where people were processed and then found their "proper place without unnecessary rehandling, arriv[ing] at the finished stock room ready to crate and ship."[51] Or, as another critic put it, the "fine intimate personal touch between patient and physician is lost completely.... The patients are overhauled like automobiles."[52] Ford himself was personally slammed—not inaccurately—as "a man of unlimited wealth and power, a man who controls a publication, a man of strong prejudices," and perhaps most damning, a man who was *not* a doctor. He was guilty of "practic[ing] medicine by proxy."[53]

Critiques of Ford's group practice approach probably attained greater publicity simply because they were attached to Ford. At least, Ford was an easier and more uncontroversial target for detractors of the approach who steered clear of critiquing the most prominent implementation of assembly-line medicine at the Mayo Clinic.

The loudness and vehemence of these critiques thus does not suggest as much as one might expect about the popularity of assembly-line medicine or its take-up. One doctor lauded the Ford Hospital's "application of factory methods to the handling of patients" for the clear improvements this systematizing would bring to hospital function.[54] Newspaper articles were equally effusive: "Everything comes in one end," said one, ahead of the Ford Hospital's planned construction in 1918, "and goes out the other," a logic that followed both "the system of nature and the modern factory."[55] To many, the assembly-line outpatient clinic appeared to be simply good, smart doctoring, and the system proved as popular at the Ford Hospital as it had at the Mayo Clinic and other places. In his own defense of this system, the Ford Hospital surgeon-in-chief Roy McClure pointed out that it was primarily through the informal, word-of-mouth marketing of "satisfied patients" that the Ford Hospital had experienced such "phenomenal growth." Over 40,000 patients, he declared, couldn't be wrong.[56]

Though those critical of assembly-line medicine dressed their critiques in a language that set assembly lines and group practice as antithetical to real care, in fact there is good reason to think that their problem with group practice was actually about its financial implications. A few years before the Ford Hospital opened, in the muckraking *American Magazine*, the prominent physician Richard Cabot both anticipated and discredited the complaints of critics like those lashing out against the Ford Hospital. Calling foul on their complaint that the group practice method would destroy the sacrosanct doctor-patient relationship, Cabot explained that though it might appear that cooperative diagnosis came at the cost of the "intimacy of the best type of private physicians and his patients," very few patients actually enjoyed this kind of relationship with their practitioners. It was a luxury item, limited only to those who could afford the exorbitant fees of the private doctor.[57]

Indeed, the vast majority of patients received their care from whomever, wherever, and whenever they could. Given that any medical intimacy was available only to the few, and given the fact that it often came at the expense of accurate diagnosis, Cabot could not see how its loss could be viewed as all that great.[58] Why pay doctors to nod sympathetically to health woes they could neither really diagnose nor treat when you could get a friend to do this for free? Among other things, it just wasn't a great value for money.

As Cabot implied—and his physician brother Hugh Cabot repeated years later—the attacks leveled against group practice, reflected in exaggerated form in critiques of the Ford Hospital, did not reflect something axiomatic about health care. They were instead a targeted marketing policy aimed at attracting back to the fold those patients wealthy enough to pay for the one thing these practitioners could promise that modern medical practitioners no longer would: a personal relationship, priced like a luxury product.[59]

In fact, the adoption of group practice at the Mayo Clinic had done little to dampen the love that medical practitioners and patients alike felt for the beloved brothers, "Doctor Will and Doctor Charlie," as they were known to patients. Indeed, in certain senses, it was just the opposite: patient processing at the Mayo Clinic was welcomed as a guarantor of full and complete "care." It was certainly viewed as a positive addition at many of the East Coast hospital heavyweights—Johns Hopkins and Cabot's own Massachusetts General Hospital, among others. In this way, at least, the attacks on group practice and the systematization of hospitals that went with it reflected an underlying and deep-rooted concern about money. And, on this score, the Ford Hospital was exceptional and its attraction of especially zealous critique understandable. For the one thing that was really "Fordist" about the Ford Hospital was its pricing structure.

A Ford Product

Though Ford's decisions were not discontinuous with those of other hospitals at the time, the rationale he gave for making these decisions was. Ford explained to all who would listen that the uniform rooms, the adherence to group practice, the closed staff were all in service to the greater goal of establishing flat fees for every service the hospital provided. Ford's frequent ghostwriter Samuel Crowther described this specifically in relation to the decision for uniform rooms: "Aside from the additional expense of attending rooms of various sizes and appointments, it would be necessary to charge each patient according to the square footage—which would at once prevent a flat rate. [Ford] wanted flat rates."[60]

Likewise, much of the appeal of group practice and a closed staff was the standardization of fees that it made possible. In the diagnostic unit, each specialist repeated a specific battery of tests for each new patient. It made sense to charge a flat fee for this kind of process, and in 1926, this stood at $13 per visit.[61]

But it wasn't only the diagnostic unit that was affected by Ford's insistence on flat rates. Everything—from room cost to treatment fees to hourly wages and salaries for workers—was set at a standard rate. In 1926, a room at the Ford Hospital reportedly cost $8 a day, including board, nursing, and newspaper delivery. Those who needed medical care during their stay at the Ford Hospital paid an additional $3 daily. Treatment prices were similarly fixed. And though costs varied from disease to disease, they did not vary from person to person—everyone paid the same.[62] Childbirth cost $75. Appendectomies were $125. And though there was slightly more wiggle room for pricing surgical procedures, they were capped at $250.[63]

The flat fee broke dramatically with established practices at the nation's hospitals, where fees were often figured after the fact, largely using an opaque and ever-shifting assessment of what a particular person could afford to pay, balanced against equipment and labor costs and the like. Those who supported the Ford Hospital decried this as an outdated business practice that allowed doctors to perpetuate the anti-modern habit of relating charges not to costs but to "what the traffic would bear."[64]

A more insidious but arguably more accurate variation was the fee-setting method used at the Mayo Clinic, which also based its prices on observed wealth. This likely protected the Mayo brothers from the kind of ostracism and critique received by those working at the Ford Hospital. As Cabot wrote,

> The fee is determined, as I understand it, by a business agent of the Mayo Clinic, who has correspondents in all parts of the country and whose object is to discover approximately the income of every patient visiting that clinic. From the figure thus obtained regarding the patient's income, the fee can be calculated upon a percentage system.[65]

Even this rather intrusive method of establishing fees was preferable, at least in the medical mind, to the flat fee.

Back in Detroit, Ford's pricing structure was met with outrage from the area's medical practitioners. The Detroit Academy of Surgery and the Wayne County Medical Society particularly lashed out at the Ford Hospital, since it disrupted the practice of assessing oversized fees to the wealthy, sometimes just as a way of making money (as Cabot pointed out) and sometimes as a way of recouping losses incurred by providing free services to the poor.

Compounding the income problems of those practitioners who felt themselves hung out to dry on the back of the Ford policies, flat fees at the Ford Hospital proved enticing not only to the middle class, at whom they were supposedly aimed, but also to the rich who, Ford opined, were relieved to see medicine adhere to the "one price system" that had become increasingly common in retail trade.[66] As a result, the economics of local medical practice had been thrown into disarray. The very poor, they argued, who could not afford to go to the Ford Hospital despite the low fees, continued to call on private practitioners. These, having lost the fees of their rich patients, found themselves without any way to recoup the losses incurred by giving away their services to the poor. They were thus reduced, they complained, to practicing medicine for free.[67]

The Ford Hospital refused to back down. Acknowledging the "rough justice" of effectively charging the wealthy for the care of the poor, it also asserted its own right to provide a service with fees based on cost. Ford explained that his flat fees had been set with the middle-class consumer in mind. "In recent years," he noted, "it has often been said that only the very rich and the very poor could obtain the best medical service." No one, it seemed, was looking out for the growing middle class. The Ford Hospital remedied this situation by adopting the revolutionary notion that one ought not to tie fees and services to what it appeared that patients could pay but instead to cost.[68]

But the more Fordist point of this flat rate was the socioeconomic equality this kind of price-fixing ostensibly marked out. Because the Ford Hospital prices were purportedly fixed so that only the most destitute would find them out of reach, (almost) anyone would be able to pay for services rendered, producing a mixing of classes that was otherwise absent from medicine. Just as all rooms should be alike, as one newspaper put it:

> It was Mr. Ford's theory that all patients should pay the same price for the same service, be they millionaires or paupers. It is true in the Henry Ford Hospital that all patients receive the same treatment and are presented with bills which represent the exact service that is rendered them. If the patient is so poor that he cannot meet his bill, it remains unpaid and the hospital takes the loss.[69]

The commitment to this efficiency-infused brand of egalitarianism tied the Ford Hospital explicitly back to the founding premise of the Ford Motor Company, which Detroit's wealthy elites despised as much as its medical elite despised the Ford Hospital.[70] And for many of the same reasons.

Breaking with the automotive tradition, in which cars were made and marketed as luxury items for the wealthy elite only, Ford set out to democratize cars and make them available to what he called the "producing class" that had previously been shut out of car ownership. This reflected Ford's view that investing in this producing—this "consumer"—class stimulated economic growth, a view that the monopoly-minded industrial capitalists, who had made their fortunes in things like coal, steel, oil, and electricity, found exceedingly alarming, both for its potential social ramifications and what they feared would be dire financial consequences for the nation.[71]

Ford was unmoved by these arguments. As he told a car dealer in 1906, the whole purpose of his plant would be to produce a car that "anyone can afford to own."[72] This "universal car," as Ford envisioned it in the years just prior to the Model T's appearance, would be affordable even for the burgeoning middle class.[73] It would, he further told the car dealer, ideally cost about $500. In addition, it would

> be cheap enough for the salaried man to buy, light enough in weight so that the cost of the upkeep, tires etc., would not be prohibitive; so simple in construction that the average man could keep it in repair, so perfect and uniform in its components that these parts would be on sale in all hardware stores and could be purchased at as low a comparative price as the parts for [a] lady's sewing machine.[74]

Ford was better than his word. In 1908, the first year the Model T car ran off the production line, it cost about $950, but by 1925, it cost only $260. This was assembly-line economics.[75] In the first few months of operation, the Ford Motor Company, operating at maximum capacity, had only been able to produce about a dozen cars. By 1914, the company was able to build a new car in under two hours. By 1925, over half of all automobiles on the road—worldwide—were Model Ts.

Ford's production model was specifically driven by the notion that refining the product was less important than perfecting the process by which it was manufactured. The product needed simply to meet the minimum requirements of being uniform, reliable, repeatable, and almost by virtue of these traits, desirable. For this reason, the Model T notoriously changed very little over its nineteen-year production run, a situation that occasioned one of Ford's many quotable quotes: "Any customer can have a car painted any color that he wants so long as it is black."[76]

The price for the Model T also reflected Ford's egalitarian stylings. Set at a rate that was "less than the traffic might have borne," Ford took the gamble that this would so enlarge his consumer base that it would more than make up for smaller profit margins per car.[77] What really mattered in this equation, and where the savings would take place, was on the factory floor. Increasing production efficiency, Ford theorized, could drive costs down enough that it would more than make up for these smaller profit margins. About cars, at least, Ford was right.

On the factory floor, Ford's commitment to the selfsame egalitarianism that drove his desire to produce cars for the producing class was also extant. This perhaps explains why Ford was so insistent on describing the trial-and-error method of creating standardized processes as unique to his own business philosophy, even though it had been circulating in efficiency circles far earlier. It must have been incredibly satisfying to credit the selfsame producing class who would buy the cars also with the innovations that made them so widely available. The Model T was a car for producers, by producers.

Working in this way against norms regarding class and social position, as well as against the very notions of how industrial capitalism was supposed to work, the Ford Motor Company offered up a "business proposition" that was simultaneously, if not more fundamentally, a "social provocation." And part of what made it so provocative was its unbelievable success, at least in the short term.[78]

It is clear that it was precisely this model that Ford eventually adopted for his hospital. To some degree sidelining his earlier hope that the hospital would implement his philosophy of health much as his sociological department had done in the 1910s, Ford instead put his stamp on the hospital as a further implementation of his vision of affordability as a means of economic enfranchisement. This was in part why Ford was so insistent that his work was not philanthropic but the home of the square deal. "Everybody pays," as one admiring description put it, but "nobody pays too much."[79] It was, as another explained, *therefore* a "Ford product."[80]

Given the analogue between the Ford Factory and hospital, it is unsurprising that it should have met with such hostility from Detroit's medical elite. They were, after all, members of the same elite class that had initially derided his cars for the populist challenge to the business convention they represented. Of course, just as he had in the business world, Ford was looking to remake medical financing by standardizing fees, lowering prices, and increasing production efficiency, all with the goal of building out medicine as a consumer good that, by virtue of its potentially huge and largely untapped market, could be made both affordable *and* profitable. The medical elite of Detroit and across the nation rejected this view, not least for the challenge it posed to medicine's conventional business logic.

The implementation of this egalitarian-suffused business philosophy, for a time so successful in the factory, did not translate well to the Ford Hospital. This is not to say that Ford didn't try. In addition to its standardized rates, the hospital paid standardized wages to help hold on to its workers. "Laborers" in the hospital—made up of everyone except doctors and upper management (who received a set salary)—were paid exactly the same as their industrial counterparts. Also, thanks to Ford's increasingly capacious portfolio of business, they received discounts on various household basics. Eleven dollars, for example, could normally purchase about a ton of coal.[81] With the Henry Ford employee discount, it bought three.[82]

Yet, despite the potential promise that rationalized health care pricing and salaries held for correcting some of the more obvious inequities of medical economics, the Ford Hospital never came close to being self-sustaining or even turning a profit in Ford's lifetime. Though the hospital did, as anticipated, attract droves of patients with its pricing structure and efficiency improvements, their numbers were simply not enough to offset the low fixed fees they paid.

The fact that the Ford Hospital stayed in business despite its unbalanced books is one of the key pieces of evidence that Ford biographers and the Ford Company's commemorative materials point to in labeling the hospital a philanthropic enterprise. Indeed, the outright charitable giving of the Ford family vis-à-vis the hospital was substantial. In addition to footing the bill for construction and making up the hospital's annual shortfall, Ford sought little to no payment for the use of the hospital grounds by the federal government and then by the city of Detroit between 1914 and 1921.[83] Ford habitually offered free service to veterans and their families when the Veterans Administration refused to pay, and he (along with his wife and his son) were well known for their willingness to step in and pay the bills for particularly needy patients, especially if they were children.[84] By 1936, a few years into the Great Depression, the Ford family had spent nearly $15 million keeping the Ford Hospital afloat.[85]

But auditing the accounting in a slightly different way points to an alternate conclusion. Ford's hospital also manifested the kind of vertical integration that served the health and wealth of the population not for its own sake but as a boon for Ford's automotive arm. Indeed, questions that turned the definition of a healthy and fit population on what it produced and consumed had become part of the discussion of how to measure the value and success of a hospital in the first place. According to one accounting, a good hospital saved 10 percent of the patients it cared for. Since "the value of human life today is estimated at $6,000," it summarized, one could easily assess the real return on investment of any hospital and weigh this against costs.[86] If Roy McClure was right that between the opening of the new building in 1921 and 1924 the Ford Hospital had seen approximately 40,000 patients, then the hospital had produced an economic benefit of at least $24 million over that same period. It had saved a population of people who could now go on living, possibly go on to purchase Ford vehicles, and perhaps more importantly, contribute to an economy that supported his efficiency methods. Perhaps the Ford Hospital was, after all, just another experiment in the selfsame art of "industrial welfare work"—this time on a massive scale—that Ford had so diligently and relentlessly implemented in his factory.

Whether this approach has currency or not, it is the case that the hospital manifested the same Fordist philosophy of spreading social mobility through affordability that his factories had. But it also made even clearer the philosophy's absolute limits. One glaring contradiction of the whole Fordist regime and its purported egalitarianism comes through the simultaneous enfranchising/disenfranchising of Ford's Black workers.

Though critics at the time chose to pick other bones, the Henry Ford Hospital did not share the integrationist ethos—if one can call it that—of the Ford Factory. Indeed, when Vivien Thomas, the famed surgical assistant and collaborator to Alfred Blalock, wrote to his sister in Detroit in 1937 with the news that he and Blalock might move their work there, she told him not to get his hopes up. The Ford Hospital, she wrote, was "lily white" and worse than "anything she had seen," even though "she had grown up in the South."[87] A 1926 survey of the hospitals of Detroit affirmed that in the preceding decade, there were no Black physicians at the Ford Hospital and no Black medical staff at all. This situation remained unchanged until the 1950s.[88]

Unfortunately, those at the Ford Hospital who filled out this survey left blank any questions about how many Black patients had been treated at the hospital in the preceding year. Though this questionnaire recorded "no" as the Ford Hospital's response to a question about whether the hospital was segregated, it also contained the unsolicited comment that Black patients "must occupy private rooms," which was a nod both to the Fordist focus on private rooms and to the dodging of segregation questions that private rooms made possible.[89] The history of the hundredth anniversary of the Henry Ford Health System offers a slightly different view. At least during the 1950s, it records, Black patients *were* segregated. They were housed in the hospital's original building: the same one Ford had decried as inefficient and anti-modern.[90]

Whatever the exact provisions made for Black patients, the clear absence of a commitment to integration in this piece of the Ford empire at least doubles down on the scholarly observation that Ford's commitment to racial equality in the factory was not ideological but opportunistic: an expedient solution to the high labor turnover that the automotive industry suffered more broadly.[91] But these were more than just ideological discontinuities. For the hospital's lack of integration only added to the more general discriminatory policies to which Detroit's Black community, vastly enlarged by Ford's equal pay policies, was subject.

Housing was by no means a singular example in this regard. Landlords would not rent and banks would not lend to the Black community, rendering the potential for mobility implicit in Ford's equal wages extremely limited.[92] Those who were able to buy a house and thus make the move out of Detroit's overcrowded Black neighborhood, Black Bottom, and into white neighborhoods were not infrequently driven out. This was something that Ossian Sweet, a prominent doctor (not at the Ford Hospital), experienced in 1925. The day he moved his family into his newly purchased house in Detroit's white East Side neighborhood was also the day he left it: a mob arrived to make it clear that Sweet was not welcome, and the violence that followed left him on trial for murder.[93]

The hospital's own exclusionary practices were part and parcel of the larger discriminatory culture that permeated Detroit at the time and a social apparatus that was geared, at best, toward segregating Black residents and, at worst, forcing them out. At one end of the spectrum, then, Ford gave Black workers access to the "new world" of "modernity" by offering them unprecedented access to jobs.[94] And at the other end, through the policies at the Ford Hospital, he closed that new world off. In this sense, the efficiency philosophy that the hospital manifested, touting affordability as a mechanism for social mobility, was quite clearly delimited: it did not, after all, cross what W. E. B. Du Bois had famously called the "color line."[95]

Conclusion

The racial capitalism built directly into the Ford empire made it clear why Black workers would not reap the benefits of the social mobility Fordism supposedly brought with it. Even if the burgeoning white middle class—those who were intended to gain from the social mobility promised—did benefit from Fordism at the Ford Hospital, Fordism at the hospital itself proved to be unsustainable. Perhaps the most obvious reason was the difficulty of applying the logic of ever-increasing production efficiency as a route to lower costs in a hospital setting. Among other things, humans were not as predictable as automobiles, nor were their parts and problems as clearly understood. The reliable improvements in efficiency year upon year that made the Ford Factory so phenomenally successful were not easily translated to health and health care.

There was also the matter of strong pushback against the Fordist model from the established medical groups of the period, for whom this shift in pricing convention reflected a disturbing disruption to the pricing methods that they, especially given their ever-growing relationship with the Carnegie and Rockefeller foundations, believed were the better solution to settling and stabilizing the turbulent medical market.[96] While it would be an overstatement to say that these forces were stronger than they had been in the automobile marketplace, it is certainly the case that in the hospital, the absence of a clear success, of the sort that Ford had enjoyed with the Model T, would have made even his staunchest supporters wary of Ford's insistence that this logic could be translated to medicine or, indeed, other settings beyond his own factory walls.

A key element that has received little attention, but also likely undermined the implementation of Ford's purportedly square deal philosophy at his hospital, was the unrest at his own company when the hospital opened. In the years between 1914, when Ford acquired the hospital, and 1921, when it finally opened, Ford's famous day wage of $5 had reached its limits; likewise, the sociological department set up to support Ford's welfare capitalism became more obviously the blunt tool of industry than an uplifting instrument of the Social Gospel. Indeed, during the years between the acquisition and the opening of the Ford Hospital, things at the Ford company changed. And so did the world—transformed not least by the experiences of World War I and the defeat of that erstwhile giant of efficiency and medical thought, Germany.

Perhaps if the Ford Hospital had opened just a decade earlier, it might have pulled medicine with it into the welfare-infused capitalism that Ford had so successfully established with his cars. Or it may be that the Great Depression changed Ford's relationship to his hospital, from one forged in the populist ethos and consumer-driven successes of his factory to one that embodied the very thing he had set out to disrupt—a model of capital investment brought to medicine by way of the Carnegie and Rockefeller foundations.

Either way, the end might not have been so different: both medicine and Fordism were ultimately recast in the 1970s as oppressive forces for many of the same reasons. Both were criticized for exemplifying what was viewed as the inexorable rise of corporate or, in the case of medicine, professional hegemony. And both were thus roundly incorporated into a trajectory beset by bad acts, bad faith, and monopolistic thinking, typified in twentieth-century medicine by the actions of the AMA, which became the major villain. Breaking somewhat with that scholarship, this chapter offers a far more granular view. In the story of the Henry Ford Hospital, there are efficiency principles implemented with varying motivations and expectations, inconstant execution, and surprising results. There are grand plans that never materialized and experiments that reverberated across the century. There are a multiplicity of competing interests and visions that shaped medicine's trajectory. And there is racial capitalism, here breaking through the artifice of efficiency-suffused egalitarianism to suggest, as it will elsewhere, that efficiency's role in constructing modern medicine comes in the particular structuring of disenfranchisement that it simultaneously accomplishes.

3

The Standard

The difference in the care of a patient in a standardized hospital from a non-standardized hospital is the difference in the feeling that a fellow had fifty years ago when he rode on an old rickety chair car on a narrow-gauge railroad and what he has today when he rides on a steel Pullman on a Chicago & Alton train coming to this Convention. . . . [It] is the difference that you experience when you see the fire wagons go by here and remember that fifty years ago they had to pull them by hand and some of you fellows were the ones that pulled them. . . . [It] is the difference you would find if you had to register at the Salvation Army headquarters tonight and you got a cot and somewhere to wash your face in the morning, but come to this fine hostelry and get the nice room and care that goes with it.—ROBERT JOLLY, MD, FACS, at the Hospital Conference of the American College of Surgeons, October 22–23, 1923

In the July 1914 issue of the monthly hospital trade journal the *Modern Hospital*, Asa Bacon, the superintendent of the Presbyterian Hospital Chicago, shared the blueprint for his newest piece of hospital technology. In loving detail, he described the workings of his "tin can crusher," a device that, as the name

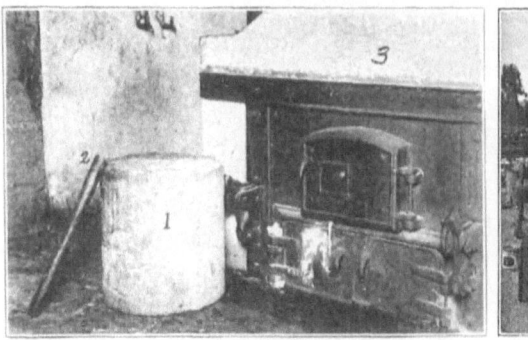 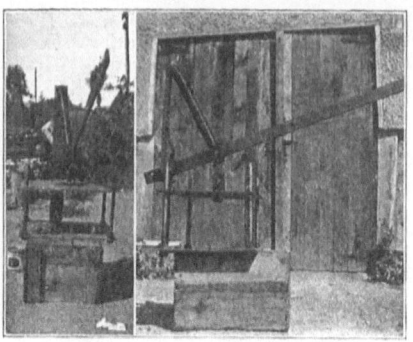

FIGURE 3.1. Competing designs for tin can crushers submitted by P. W. Behrens and Asa Bacon to the Home-Made Hospital Appliances section of *Modern Hospital* approximately four months apart in 1914.

suggested, crushed tin cans. Bacon helpfully illustrated his description with a photo of the machine, with numbers identifying its component parts. Figure 1: a concrete block. Figure 2: a "can smasher" (to the layperson, this might look like a length of pipe). Figure 3: a garbage burner, present for unspecified reasons, since the crushed cans were carted off rather than incinerated. He then laid out clear instructions for those who needed more than visual cues: "Lay a can on the block. Hit it once or twice with the smasher, and it becomes flat instead of round."[1]

Though underwhelming in appearance, purpose, and complexity, Bacon's particular invention was not an unusual contribution to the journal's "Home-Made Hospital Appliances" column, which featured ideas sent in from hospital administrators and medical practitioners across the country. Indeed, just four months later, the feature published a challenge to Bacon's can crusher: the "can masher," the brainchild of one P. W. Behrens, the superintendent of the Lake Forest University (figure 3.1). The masher was presented as having certain advantages over the crusher. Because it consisted of a giant lever with a plate attached, it required less in the way of human labor. And because the plate was quite large, it was possible to mash two cans at a time. "One or more cans are set under the plate and the powerful lever is brought down upon them." The satisfying result: "very flat" cans.[2]

Of course, a solution to the superabundance of empty tin cans was not the only thing on the minds of readers. In the first months after the column's introduction, the *Modern Hospital* was flooded with mail from enterprising hospital workers around the country who sent in descriptions, designs, and photos.[3]

More recognizably clinical innovations like automatic infant feeders, sterilizers, wheeled objects of all sorts, and "open-air" beds for tubercular patients joined kitchen steam tables, parcel, library, and food trucks, ventilation system improvements, and other innovations meant to improve the built environment of the hospital more generally.

Though some contributions to the column seemed to have utility in only narrow contexts, each featured idea was selected by the editors for its potential to become *the* design for that purpose that all hospitals adopted. Indeed, as the editors explained, the purpose of the column was to turn local innovation into national standards. If enough people read about and like the nominated invention, it might then be replicated at other hospitals across the country. Full-scale adoption was then only a matter of capturing the attention of the "commercial folks" whose manufacturing expertise would transform this custom design into a standard artifact with reliable uniformity and wide distribution. What had once been a design specific to a particular individual or hospital would become the industry standard.[4]

In the case of competing designs, as with the can mashers, this process was to be one of the survival of the fittest, as determined by consensus. Only one can-crushing prototype could catch the fancy of hospitals across the country, the column editors presumed. Would it be Bacon's easily built but more labor-intensive smasher? Or Behrens's more complex but more powerful masher? To the victor would go the spoils: widespread acclaim as having set the new standard for can-flattening technology.

Submissions to the column came hard and fast, with some contributors seeming to take a rather scattershot approach, sending in designs and ideas for just about anything that crossed their minds. Bacon himself maintained a constant presence, with proposals that ranged from a fully operational hospital call system to an electric fan modified into a shear sharpener, to one of his more dubious inventions—a decorative "quiet zone" sign designed to "relieve the ugliness" of such fixtures in hospital neighborhoods.[5] That his innovation turned out to be the planting of flowers in a trough beneath the sign, which was otherwise unchanged, and that the accompanying image further clarified that the trough of flowers in question was so small and inconsequential as to be practically invisible in the photo did not seem to trouble the column editors, who commented that they had great hope for the "more luxurious growth" of the plants Bacon foresaw for his sign's future.[6]

Such was the enthusiasm for invention and standardization that suffused medicine over the first decades of the twentieth century. Though the "Home-Made Hospital Appliances" column eventually disappeared from the *Modern*

Hospital, the method of standardizing objects that it explicitly espoused presented a snapshot of one critical trajectory for medical standardization, in which not just appliances but hospitals, medical sects, and individual practitioners of all kinds competed for the prize of setting the "standard." Many thought this process would best take place on a fair and open playing field, with the modern medicine that emerged presumably one that its constituent parts had democratically adopted. The less popular medical possibilities that were not picked up as standard would naturally slough off and disappear, drummed out of business by the more successful design of their counterparts.

This trajectory from innovation to standardization had its doubters, not least among them the industrial efficiency experts. As Frank Gilbreth disapprovingly put it, this trajectory for standardization had only yielded an "insanity for inventing."[7] One example from medicine was the practice—common among surgeons—of designing and then working exclusively with their own instruments. Each surgeon claimed the primacy of his own stitch cutter over those of his peers, even though it typically deviated as much from a colleague's as Bacon's "decorative" quiet sign did from its reportedly uglier counterparts. There could be little consensus among those who brought such a rigidly individualistic approach to their work.

As Gilbreth explored the matter for his study of hospital efficiency in the 1910s, his interviewees bemoaned the chaos wreaked by this practice. Nurses explained that these personal surgical "tools" (to maintain an industrial coherence, Gilbreth insisted on using the term "tool" rather than "instrument") were often indistinguishable from each other in function. One nurse complained to Gilbreth that she was "in trouble all the time" with a surgeon who insisted on the exclusive use of the 150 instruments he had invented. The sheer number of his tools, added to the fact that they were "so nearly alike the other instruments in the operating room," left her with no hope of keeping them straight.[8]

Others told similar tales, with many reporting that proprietary instruments were quite often paired with exacting demands about operating room setup and etiquette. One nurse knew "five hundred ways to set up [an] operating room," but what was worse was that she was never told in advance which setup any surgeon preferred. "I have not the remotest idea of what the doctor wants until he gets in this room," she despaired to Gilbreth.[9] Both scenarios created a colossal waste of labor and time.

For many, if not all, industrial efficiency experts, it became clear that far from leading to standardization, invention—especially the invention of more things that did the same tasks as objects that already existed—was the mother of inefficiency. And even when something like the tin can crusher came along to alleviate the problem of storing spent cans, it was not clear that the extra labor and time required to operate it would have a reasonable efficiency trade-off.[10]

Those outside the medical world were spared much concern over the mechanics of tin can mashing or the woeful and counterproductive power dynamics of the operating room. But both practitioners and efficiency experts realized that medical standardization had a vital public-facing value—one that would bestow a market advantage on whoever could sell their own standards as a consumer good. At this moment, the medical marketplace was flooded with a dizzying number of options, with osteopaths, chiropractors, naturopaths, eclectics, and other brands of practitioner all sharing space with the allopathic (today's mainstream) practitioners. Consumers were spoiled for choice but hard-pressed, as standardization's proselytizers saw it, to make especially meaningful distinctions between the various alternatives.[11] Establishing and selling a standard would have market-shaking benefits—the problem was figuring out where standards would come from and how they could be agreed.

This chapter explores this push and pull of standardization at the American College of Surgeons. Often overlooked, in part because of the historical prioritization of the activities of the American Medical Association's far more autocratic tendencies in the establishment of standards, the College was in fact the consummate medical standardizing body of the early twentieth century. Founded in 1913 for the rather amorphous purpose of "elevat[ing]the standard of surgery" (a charge that it had shared with many other surgical organizations of its era), its signature effort was undoubtedly the standardization of hospitals.[12] Indeed, the Joint Commission, the primary accrediting body for health organizations in the United States, draws a straight line from the American College of Surgeons' efforts to standardize hospitals from 1910 onward to its own accrediting efforts today.[13]

Though at first blush the College's standardizing efforts seem to map onto the rather more generic script of standardization through autocratic imposition often assigned to medicine's history, its standardization programs actually reveal the far more complex process by which standards were understood and designed in this period. Tied up implicitly in questions about how far the more populist mode of standardization could take medicine—as described especially well in the early attempts at object standardization in the *Modern Hospital*—and what the democratic form of standard medicine ought to be, the standardization activities at the College describe the politics of standardization more broadly as they were being hashed out over the efficiency-suffused 1910s and 1920s.

Standardization

Standardization, as many sociologists have explained, can take many different forms, but its greatest goal is commonly considered to be the production of uniformity.[14] And uniformity can be powerful. As Susan Leigh Star and Geoffrey Bowker point out in their classic text on the subject, standards make things work together over different communities and modes of practice and across time and space. Standardized building materials, standardized sizes of nails and screws, standardized wall outlets with standardized voltages of electricity coming out of them, standardized educational curricula and testing, standardized languages and spelling, standardized water, electric, sewage and gas system supplies, standardized trains and buses are just some of the individual constituent parts that make our lives function smoothly.[15]

In the context of the political history of efficiency, more often than not, standards get a bad rap. In the factory, standardization often features as part of a larger imposition of technocracy and the shifting fortunes of industrial worker autonomy and agency. Standard-setting thus accomplished two key goals: it displaced the experiential knowledge of workers with more arbitrary—but supposedly scientifically acquired—guidelines set by a new and extensive managerial class, and it used these standards as a way to measure and perhaps even to discipline workers and their work.[16]

Of course, there were the paths to standardization that were coterminous with autocracy and monopoly. Indeed, these are probably some of the best known: corporations that acquired such size and heft in the marketplace that they were able to set industry standards according to their own interests.[17] This was the path we generally assign to monopolistic behemoths of the age, like John D. Rockefeller's Standard Oil, infamous in its own time thanks to Ida Tarbell's famous 1904 muckraking exposé revealing the illegal and nefarious means by which it acquired its size.[18] But even as the company was vilified for its illegal practices and ultimately prosecuted under the Sherman Antitrust Act, Standard Oil's arbitrary standard-setting was not—at least theoretically—a terrible solution for consumers to the chaos of the industrial marketplace. Indeed, as its market share rose over the 1870s, from 4 percent to a whopping 90 percent, the price passed on to consumers fell, from 25 cents a gallon to just under 10 cents.[19]

The nineteenth century embrace of standardization found powerful expression in medicine. It was at this time that doctors began to categorize pathologies, grouping what otherwise might have been viewed as disparate and independently addressed symptoms into a single disease taxonomy with a set of clear qualities and characteristics.[20] The efficiency-suffused early twentieth century gave this still incomplete transformation new impetus. As the major medical efficiency figure Abraham Flexner explained, the new "science" of management was *the* science that revolutionized medicine; the efforts of humans to "purify, extend, and organize their knowledge of the world in which they live" comprised science in its purest form. Although laboratories or technologies might be able to augment these activities—using microscopy, for example—their presence was not a guarantor of scientific activity, nor did they provide the skills required to transform medicine. These would take place instead through the science of efficiency.[21]

Flexner knew what he was talking about, even if his words seem unintuitive to us now. In the hands of the efficiency zealot and surgeon Ernest Amory Codman, for example, the mere act of compiling the different characteristics and qualities of bone tumors from across the medical landscape into a single registry yielded a clear set of symptoms and clinical qualities that permitted doctors to better distinguish between malignant and benign tumors. It also offered a clear sense of therapeutic dos and don'ts, a list derived directly from tabulating reports of treatments and carefully following up on their outcomes. Exemplifying the basic sense that the acts of standardizing, organizing, and codifying were not activities done after knowledge was already made but instead themselves knowledge-making activities, Codman's registry manifested a critical component of the "science" of medicine as efficiency practitioners generally understood it. This was a science capable of revolutionizing health care—*modernizing* it—simply by virtue of the outsized contributions that organization made in the development of new information. Far more than laboratory science, which, according to another commentator, had fallen away since medicine's "golden year[s]" of scientific discovery around the turn of the century, the science of standardization promised real, lasting, and continuous results.[22]

Though uniformity has in retrospect seemed to be the presumptive goal of medical standardization, in fact it was in many cases neither the only goal nor the most important one. For Codman himself, a prominent goal of standardization was *also* the abolition of medical elitism, to be replaced with—on both the professional and consumer side—a critical egalitarianism. This was made clear in some of his showier attacks on the profession, including a cartoon featuring a "goose-ostrich" meant to represent those hapless patients of Boston's wealthy Back Bay neighborhood who paid for often-unnecessary surgeries with their giant golden eggs (figure 3.2). Possibly more productively (or at least less snarkily), his standardization ideals led him to open his own small ten-bed hospital. It was an institution that he dedicated to operating according to standardization principles, and not accidentally, it was located just down

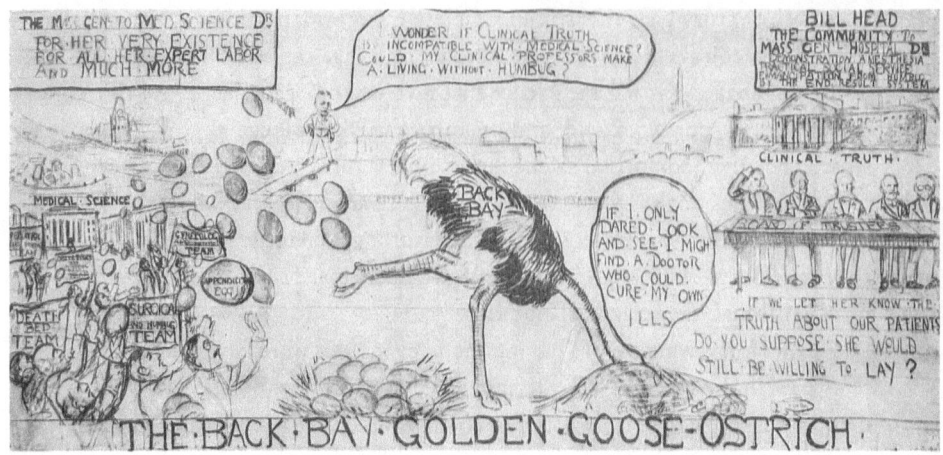

FIGURE 3.2. One of Codman's more audacious publicity events for his medical efficiency fixes featured a cartoon titled "The Back Bay Golden Goose-Ostrich," produced by his friend Philip Hale. Codman unveiled it at the Suffolk District Medical Society's Meeting for the Discussion of Hospital Efficiency at the Boston Medical Library on January 6, 1915. The cartoon offered in caricature and metaphor the conspiracy of hospital trustees, physicians, surgeons, the Harvard Medical School, and the public that Codman felt his efficiency interventions would expose and remove. Ernest Amory Codman, "Preface," in *The Shoulder: Rupture of the Supraspinatus Tendon and Other Lesions in or about the Subacromial Bursa*, 1934, xxvi.

the road from his powerful former employer, the Massachusetts General Hospital (MGH). Though the hospital could not really compete with the resources of the giant MGH, Codman hoped to use his hospital to demonstrate how his standardized system of outcome measurement, when applied to all surgeons equally, could identify those with true ability and those whose appointments had come as a result of nepotism or politics. He felt his hospital could in this way deliver a square, reasonably priced, and reliable surgical deal to the general public.[23] And he hoped that medicine would follow suit, measuring its outcomes in order to ensure transparency with the public.

This was very close to the idea of standards that Frank Gilbreth expounded when interviewed for an article in the *American Magazine*, where he explained that he had taken on his work in medical efficiency in large part to demonstrate that medicine, like every other type of work, was merely a set of learned practices, subject to all the same laws as the practices of every other kind of work. To Gilbreth, the perception that medicine was a "high-brow" occupation represented a misunderstanding that conflated class with skill. In fact, he told the interviewer, the assembly line worker was just as skillful as the highly esteemed surgeon in the egalitarian eyes of the efficiency expert.[24]

This view certainly directed Gilbreth's conversation with two collaborators from the New York Hospital, the surgeons Frederick Bancroft and Eugene Pool, whom he invited to help him apply efficiency methods with the goal of standardizing surgical procedures. One output of their efforts was a two-page document, on which the surgeons broke down the routine appendectomy procedure into discrete, delineated steps. With these components explicitly listed, Gilbreth observed, *anybody* with the right tools, pointed to roughly the right area of the peritoneum and with a modicum of training in surgical motions, could now perform an appendectomy.[25]

The egalitarian stylings of medical standardization were clear at the *Modern Hospital*, too, where the journal's "Home-Made Hospital Appliances" columnists espoused the view that standardization brought more than the boon of uniformity. Where the key agent to an object's standardization was its popularity and subsequent adoption by a majority of consumers, standardization naturally relied on the collaborative efforts of those who actually needed and used the products to both innovate and select its final form.[26]

That standardization held such autocratic and democratic tendencies at the same time is significant, but important too is the utilitarian significance that industrial efficiency experts assigned to it. Defying the notion that standardization was fundamentally about the achievement of uniformity, they suggested that standardization would do something like its opposite: foster innovation. Even as some condemned the current mania for invention, as well as the method of standardizing that arose from this mania, efficiency experts saw standards themselves as conducive to a more organized process of invention. As one *Modern Hospital* contributor put it, in the subtitle to a far blander-sounding article on hospital organization: "organization was not a fetish, not a mechanical figure, but a flexible, living thing, by which all forces are marshaled to achievement."[27]

In this sense, standards were very much a means to an end. They offered a stopping point that forced organizations or standardizing bodies to take stock of where things stood: to assess, summarize, and consolidate those practices either across or within work settings and then to innovate from there to achieve the next standard. As the patriarch of industrial efficiency Frederick Winslow Taylor explained in his famous *Principles of Scientific Management*, standardization was a never-ending process, beginning with the almost-arbitrary setting of a standard and continuing through an evolution of standards, each improving on and displacing the previous. It was fundamentally about change, not stasis.[28]

True to his garrulous form, Gilbreth more colorfully reaffirmed this view at his intimate "standardization conference," as he called it, with the same New York surgeons who had helped him produce the beginnings of the standardized appendectomy. Standards "in no way impl[ied] perfection," he explained. Indeed, arriving at an initial standard should entail little more than jotting down current practices: "the best," as Gilbreth put it, that "you can do quickly." The real work of the standard was in its establishment of a baseline from which medical innovators might innovate. Gilbreth offered a transportation metaphor for his surgical conference attendees:

> You may be going to California in an automobile, and the main road is so bad that you take another road. If you don't keep in mind the location of the other road, you are in a bad fix, but, if you do remember, you can deviate as far as you want. Standards are only base lines to measure from. Ask him why he does deviate. I want to have tremendous standardization, and then I am willing you shall deviate as far as you want to.[29]

Standards should not be easy to change, continued Gilbreth, because this would be no better than the more populist model of standardization that Gilbreth hoped to displace. But standards should also be adaptable, because the most important goal of standardization was that standards would, through the innovation they inspired—the "side roads" of Gilbreth's metaphor—constantly improve on themselves.

Gilbreth's standardization methodology evinced the need to somehow forge a path between populist methods of standardization, which sometimes only fueled the same mania for invention that they were meant to resolve, and the autocratic methods, which heavy-handedly imposed standards from above.

This was indeed the problem that perplexed Flexner, possibly the best-known figure in the history of medical standardization, in the years prior to the work that would make him famous: the Carnegie Foundation study of medical education. Flexner was an educational reformer first and foremost, and in his early work, he had seen exactly how standardization could go wrong. On the one hand, the imposition of standards from above had obligated students to churn through an unchanging body of classic literature and languages, regardless of the relevance of things like ancient Greek to modern life.[30] On the other hand, in an overcorrection to this "aristocratic" and "European" model of education (intended largely only to maintain class distinctions, Flexner asserted), he had seen the proliferation of electives . . . now pressed into service as standards. The educational system they produced was so free-form that it was difficult to know what exactly distinguished an educated person from an uneducated one.[31]

A similar problem was brewing at the *Modern Hospital*. As much as the editor of "Home-Made Hospital Appliances" envisioned a democratic process for standardization, it is not clear whether there was ever a clear preference among the readership for one object over another. More problematically, showcasing proprietary objects seemed to simply breed more proprietary objects. Without a large-scale enterprise—whether a manufacturer or a standardizing body—to choose one standard and enforce it, the people themselves seemed content instead to do just the opposite: they would just keep on inventing.

As Flexner and others observed, the real stakes around standardization were emblematic of the larger problems of redefining American democracy during this period. Americans were uniquely averse to the autocratic imposition of standards; indeed, Flexner habitually referenced the Revolutionary War as a conceptual break from the autocratic standardization that he saw as characteristic of European empires. But at the same time, the rampant populism of the nineteenth century had not produced a suitable alternative. In this sense, standardization was a lightning rod for anxieties about American democracy vis-à-vis the "aristocratic" values that he saw at work in the political and cultural structures of Europe. Done incorrectly, its result would be not just disorganization and disunity but elitism, classicism, and social immobility. Done well, as Flexner explained, it might create truly democratic structures that held the key to equal opportunity. When all people, no matter their social position, were held to the same standards, then those who were truly capable—no matter their social class—would inevitably rise to the top.[32]

What standardizers were learning, of course, was that standards could not be organically constructed simply through a process of popular consensus. Actually making standards that stuck instead required standardizing bodies of sufficient size, authority, and legitimacy. On this measure, there was an important distinction to be made between organizations that acquired their power in ways that looked illegitimate—like Standard Oil—and those like Andrew Carnegie's US Steel, which the trustbuster and Supreme Court justice Louis Brandeis described as having come by its size by virtue of its true embrace of efficiency.[33] Both may have passed along a key measure of standardization to consumers—reduced prices—but whereas Standard Oil posed an existential and material threat to democracy because of the process by which it acquired the size needed to standardize, US Steel did not.[34] The real-time costs to democracy that Standard Oil posed were read not just in terms of the corruption by which it gained its position, but also in terms of the marketplace insecurities that its machinations introduced, along with the company's growing political power.[35]

By the late 1910s, medical organizations keen to standardize now had plenty of examples to observe and several important guidelines to follow. To start, standardization was a beginning point, not an end—a path toward a "one best way," as Gilbreth called it, but not the one best way itself. Next, standardization would not work if the standardizing entity did not have the political heft or sheer economic size to impose its standards, yet such pull was safest when acquired legitimately. Finally, and most important for the work of the American College of Surgeons, effective standardization must feel democratic, though what democracy actually entailed was something that was to be simultaneously worked out as standardizers went along.

These were the challenges confronting the American College of Surgeons (ACS) as it began its own standardizing efforts in 1913. As the physician commentator H. B. Young put it that same year, repeating in many ways the same concerns from outside medicine, the American public would be "suspicious of anything that smacks of self-constituted authority." After all, it was self-constituted authority in the form of monarchy that had caused the "express disavowal by our forefathers" and eventually the "separation of the two peoples."[36] For the ACS to move forward with its modernization project, then, it had to do two apparently opposing things at the same time. For practical reasons, it had to establish its own authority. But to avoid violating a basic American principle, it also could *not* establish its own authority, or at least look like it had done so.[37]

This is a balance the ACS struck remarkably effectively. Understanding the need to acquire cultural capital, the ACS went out of its way to make itself—out of nothing—into a standardizing heavyweight. At the same time, it skillfully avoided becoming the sort of autocratic force that Standard Oil was. Navigating in this way between the poles of egalitarianism and autocracy, the ACS standardization story does not just articulate one instantiation of medical standardization—it demonstrates the competing ideological, political, and economic pressures for most standardizing entities over this efficiency period.

The American College of Surgeons

While undoubtedly best known for its hospital standardization program, the story the ACS tells about itself begins with the standardization of surgeons. In this narrative, the College was the brainchild of the Chicago surgeon Franklin Martin, a charismatic contributor to surgical education. Martin had founded a journal in 1905 called *Surgery, Gynecology and Obstetrics*, renamed the *Bulletin of the American College of Surgeons* in 1916 when it became the organization's official mouthpiece. In 1910, Martin joined with his colleague John Murphy to produce the first Clinical Congress of North America, an educational meeting with a strong "show and tell" vibe—live surgeries, with livelier commentary. By 1913, the congress had led to a new professional organization, the American College of Surgeons.

Like many institutions, the College dedicated itself to the vague goal of improvement in its field. It set about doing this, however, by crafting a discrete set of surgical standards and then using these to distinguish "real" surgeons from regular, run-of-the-mill physicians.[38] In return, successful candidates would pay a fee to belong to the organization and then be allowed to string the coveted letters FACS (fellow of the American College of Surgeons) behind their names.[39] These letters would be the assurance the public needed, the College thought, of the aptitude and proper training of each practitioner.

The need for such an organization, according to the ACS and its supporters, lay in the fact that at the time of its founding, any licensed medical practitioner was also qualified to practice surgery, whether or not the practitioner had ever done any training in surgery before. Since there was no way to meaningfully evaluate the differences between practitioners, a chaotic combination of personality, prices, and reputation dictated which surgeons were "good" and which were not.

The College's imposition of a standard, then, was specifically about defining and evaluating surgeons. And though there were rumblings that state licensing agencies ought to be doing this work, it was of course something of a truism that medical practitioners preferred to set these standards themselves.[40] As J. M. T. Finney, the first president of the ACS, put it, in an effort to convince the American Medical Association (AMA) to support the new organization:

> It would be shameful to delegate these functions to another, to have them usurped by the state, as will surely be the case through failure on the part of the profession, by reason of professional politics or petty jealousies and misunderstandings, to do what it is clearly its own duty to do.[41]

Not unsurprisingly, critics recognized in this standardization effort the same kind of ring-fencing that Flexner's report on medical education would also engage in—the imposition of a system designed by "a certain set of men to brand as incompetent, by refusing them admission, others as competent as themselves."[42] Others questioned the College's intention to displace the state as the proper authority to license medical practice. As one critic breathlessly put it, "The rank and file of general practitioners will bitterly resent any legislative disturbances that threaten to rob their licenses of the right to practice any branch of medicine to which their tastes, their talents and their opportunities may attract them."[43]

For many doctors, the idea that a large, elite cadre of surgeons might band together, call themselves a "college," and then dictate who *else* could become a surgeon based on a gatekeeping system that they had devised was something to worry over. It was not that they felt standardization was a negative force; rather, the worry was that the organization behind it might grow into an unstoppable autocratic force, should the standardization of surgery be successful.[44] After all, those who founded the ACS were already a part of society's "highbrow," as Gilbreth had put it, and structurally they seemed particularly well poised to confuse wealth, power, and status for surgical prowess.[45]

The College's initial plan did nothing to placate these critics. To quickly achieve the size and heft within the profession that would begin the process of its legitimation as a standardizing entity, the ACS enacted a plan of quick growth. The five hundred most prominent surgeons that the founders could think of, consisting primarily of those who were prominent because they practiced in large cities at "important universities" or were members of prominent surgical societies, were declared to have automatically met the standard and became fellows.[46] Others "whose surgeonship" could be proved by "credentials" were also automatically approved for fellowship. Ultimately, the ranks of fellows accepted without having to meet any technical requirements swelled to two thousand, comprised of what the College described as "the fittest morally, technically and surgically."[47] Though the College thus quickly achieved a surgical footing that it might have otherwise taken years to acquire, it was not a great look for an organization that insisted that its brand was, in fact, an even-handed meritocracy.[48]

Still, the tactic served its purpose. Suddenly two thousand strong, the ACS immediately gained a large foothold among prominent surgeons and quickly seemed integral to the field of surgery. Everybody who was anybody was already a fellow. Anybody who wanted to be somebody had better be one, too.

Once a market for a fellowship had been achieved, the ACS implemented an examination for those not automatically inducted—essentially anyone not already inhabiting an elite surgical position.[49] Candidates were required to show that they had at least five years of special training in surgery and that they practiced *only* surgery (there was some leeway for those who lived in smaller cities and had to also practice medicine in order to survive financially). Candidates also had to sign a pledge promising not to split fees. This was the controversial process of kickbacks on referral, and it was the College's signature "moral" requirement, to which all signed on (though not all, later reports showed, felt bound by this requirement).

In addition, candidates to the College were obligated to send along the "history or records of fifty consecutive major operations performed by himself," fifty more abstracts of operations for which the candidate had at least served as assistant, and references from surgical mentors and colleagues. In certain cases, where a candidate had not attended one of the accredited medical schools, a technical exam might also be necessary. Finally, there was the fee: $100 to be paid "within thirty days after notification of election," and an additional $25 due annually for the next four years, for a total of $200. Candidates could choose to pay all at once upon election.[50]

In practical terms, critics of this process felt that these supposed merit-based criteria were prejudicial and a matter of unequal enfranchisement. To work in a place that kept the kind of records the College asked for was already to presume an institutional recordkeeping regime that was, as the College itself would later admit, explicitly lacking in most hospitals. To have $100 floating around presumed a more lucrative salary than many who worked in smaller communities would earn. To have had the kind of education the ACS required was to dismiss any surgeon from other medical sects or the solo practitioner who had, for want of opportunity but not necessarily ambition or talent, attended a subpar medical university and then learned surgical practice in situ. In a nation that prided itself on democracy and the right to self-determination, they asked, how could an institution that curtailed these democratic possibilities in medical terms be credible and legitimate?[51]

A critical addendum to this point, and one that critics also pointed out in response to Flexner's 1910 audit of medical schools, was the geographic and social implications for those lacking the resources to apply for fellowship. If this standard held, and only those with FACS behind their names could practice surgery, surely the impact would be felt most in communities where resources were too scarce for a physician to become a fellow. For those communities where there was only one practitioner of any sort, of which there were many in the 1910s, the ultimatum that the practitioner become a member of the College or never again practice surgery was worse than impractical. It was potentially life-threatening.[52]

In this sense, the ACS seemed to amplify the already latent and sometimes quite explicit antidemocratic tendencies in American medicine. This was not a correction but a reification of how entirely and unapologetically un-American American medicine was becoming.[53] In a country that had been founded explicitly on the tenets of "representative democracy," could or should "the people" in general, and the medical and surgical professions more specifically, stand for the kind of "self-constituted authority" that the American College of Surgeons represented?[54]

One editorial worried, just as H. B. Young had before, that the College was exactly the kind of institution that the "separation . . . from our Anglo-Saxon brothers across the sea" had necessitated. If the College set standards by pure dictate, it should have no place in American medical or public life as long as the citizens of the United States—represented in this case by the country's surgical and medical practitioners—still believed in the value of their own American and democratic birthright. In its rhetorical instantiation, this was not just a matter of medicine. And it was decidedly not a matter of science. It was a matter, and an urgent one at that, of what would become of the United States as a nation if it lost its grip on its own founding tenets.[55]

A colorful critic of the ACS in this vein was the editor of the *California State Journal of Medicine*, Philip Mills Jones, who penned a series of castigating articles during the College's first year. Jones was especially attentive to what he viewed as the organization's superfluous embellishments, mercilessly mocking the pretentious features that it had borrowed directly from its transatlantic royal equivalent and suggesting that these alone sufficed as evidence that the College was decidedly and determinedly undemocratic. About the FACS designation, he suggested a variety of other, more fitting acronyms drawn from alternate names that he came up with: the "American Royal Surgical Emporium" was one; the "American Surgical Society" was another. Both provided letters that he felt would "string out behind one's name quite nicely."[56]

In another piece, he reported the news that the College had chosen a "costume." Priced at $11.90, this ceremonial outfit included a gown of "navy-blue mohair" with a "scarlet velvet facing five inches wide extend[ing] down the neck and down each side of the front." It came with a cap, he added, made "of same material as Gown with scarlet tassel."[57] Seeing in these extravagant accoutrements clear evidence of the College's less than egalitarian purposes, Jones sounded the alarm that the College's talk of being merit-based and democratic was merely rhetorical cover for medical aristocracy trooping around in fancy dress. When their fine robes fell away, he added for maximum effect, it would be revealed that these were merely "ordinary doctors who incise and suture and puncture for a living."[58]

Jones traced the source of his suspicions about the College's activities to its founders, Franklin Martin and John B. Murphy. Indeed, his distaste for the College was fed by his intense dislike of these two individuals, whose sole collective strength, he felt, was in that most taboo of medical activities, "advertising."[59] During the first decade of the twentieth century, they had each worked to establish what Jones felt were self-serving audiences: in 1905 Martin had started the journal *Surgery, Gynecology and Obstetrics*, which, unlike many journals of the day, was edited by surgeons themselves and functioned to police the line between the true "surgeon" and the dangerous dilettante. Murphy, meanwhile, had been running "wet clinics"—live surgical demonstrations—at Mercy Hospital in Chicago. These clinics were so popular that by 1912, the doctor's secretary-stenographer transcribed each session for publication. Six times a year for several years, an illustrated, verbatim account of each event went to press under the title *The Surgical Clinics of John B. Murphy, MD, at Mercy Hospital, Chicago*.

By 1910, Murphy and Martin had combined forces to introduce the Clinical Congress of North America, a series of wet clinics that ultimately displaced Murphy's and that culled its attendees from the rolls of Martin's readers. Like Murphy's clinics, these congresses were extremely popular. In that first year, which offered something of an exemplar for the congresses that would follow, Martin hoped to attract just two hundred surgeons to Chicago for a two-week event. Thirteen hundred surgeons registered. By 1913, at the fourth clinical congress in Washington, DC, at which the American College of Surgeons was officially formed, more than four thousand surgeons registered for what was now a much anticipated one-week whirlwind exhibition of surgical skill. It was at the 1912 iteration of this event, in New York City, that Codman reported having been appointed the chair of the hospital standardization committee for the yet to be incorporated new entity, the American College of Surgeons.

These congresses were supposed to be pedagogical in focus, but here too Jones had his doubts. Acquiring anything like the educational experiences Martin and Murphy promised for the event seemed logistically improbable. This was not just because venues overflowed with surgeons as eager to hobnob as they were to see their more famous peers dig into someone's anatomy. Even under the best possible circumstances, Jones guessed, it was unclear that seeing a procedure performed *once* really was that educational in the first place. If surgery was in great need of higher educative standards, as Martin claimed, surely the solution was not to be found in amassing hundreds of surgeons in one room on the off chance they would be able to catch a glimpse of some surgical procedure being taught, remember it perfectly, and then go home and replicate it.[60]

In Jones's view, the congresses, the College, and indeed the whole venture of surgical standardization were part of a monopolistic exercise supported by an elaborate and clever marketing campaign that wrapped the College up in a veneer of merit and popular democracy. In this vein, the goal indeed was to generate enough celebrity power between Murphy and Martin so that when they called to action, surgeons would want to fall into line. In both the College and the congresses before it, Jones saw a desire to seize hold of the medical profession, to define its values, and to reshape it according to the judgments of this cadre of surgical elites. These were not the people, the institution, or the values—elitism, advertising, celebrity, and thinly veiled autocracy—that ought to guide medical reform.[61]

The ACS was well aware of these kinds of critiques, and it worked hard both to position itself—and in fact to fulfill its obligations—as a "merit-based" organization. It also went to great lengths to insist that its values were those of a "popular democracy," peppering descriptions of its intentions and actions with words that emphasized this inclusivity. It had "a membership based on efficiency rather than an exclusive aristocracy based on position," it insisted at one point.[62] And it was, as one ACS spokesperson put it, an organization that was "young, but vigorous, virile, democratic, free from all entangling alliances, willing, ready and eager to perform...."[63] It was also a group wholeheartedly dedicated to helping the "physician from the small town" (provided that said physician was "honest").[64]

And in fact, the way the ACS executed its surgical standardization efforts did seem, at least to some degree, to follow up this rhetoric with real practical application. Some of the critical comments about its potentially proprietary nature were assuaged by what turned out indeed to be its real commitment to relatively widespread fellowship. Applicants, even from smaller communities, were regularly admitted to fellowship, and occasionally fellowship fees were waived, reduced, or negotiated. While in its structure and function, its policies still smacked of a kind of arbitrariness and a questionably grounded authority, in practice, the College managed to appease all but the most stubborn of its critics, paving the way for fellowship even for those who stood on the outskirts of the medical mainstream.

In large part, the College's success in this area likely stemmed from the general agreement that standardization was a good, even vital, part of medicine's modernization. Thus, the real question for the College had never been whether to go forward with standardization. It was only about how to do so in a way that allowed it to acquire the "self-constituted" authority it needed to effectively establish its standardization program while also demonstrating to the "rank and file of general practitioners of medicine and surgery and of aspiring specialists (and very many of both of these classes do excellent surgical work)" why the College's program was in their interests.[65] That is, it needed what most standardizing programs also aspired to: an autocratic agency that delivers the outcomes of meritocracy and democracy through standardization.

And it worked. The surgical standardization program accelerated, and perhaps more importantly, the ACS established itself as a reliable and relatively benign figure in standardization. It was perhaps not as democratic as the populist "Home-Made Hospital Appliances" column, but neither was it the elitist autocratic behemoth that Jones thought it would become. Still, its standardization efforts were only starting with surgeons, with its next mission to be the standardization of the hospitals of the United States and Canada. Whether hospitals were simply the logical next step or the main prize all along depends on who was telling the story.

Hospital Standardization

In the unusual autobiographical preface to his late-in-life study of the anatomy of the shoulder, Codman gave his own version of the founding of the ACS, featuring different actors and different goals. In his telling, the goal had *always* been hospital standardization, something he knew because he was there at its true beginning.[66] As he told it, the American College of Surgeons began as a germ of an idea in 1910, during a transatlantic visit that he and a small society of American surgeons made to their "British confreres" at the Royal College of Surgeons in England.

In a hansom cab on the way back to London, Codman and the American surgeon Edward Martin had talked about the growing interest in starting an American equivalent to the Royal College of Surgeons. And as their travels continued, the two traded ideas about the possible mission of this new college. Given that there were already a number of surgical organizations in the United States, they agreed that the addition of another organization would have to be carefully justified.

As it turned out, neither Codman nor Martin was interested in a new surgical organization per se, but each saw the benefit of an organization that would serve to standardize medicine more generally. The difficulty really was in creating the right organization, with the proper clout and legitimacy within medicine, to get this work done. Martin, obsessed with the idea of hospital standardization, and Codman, obsessed with the idea of outcome-based standards, hit on the idea that "an American College of Surgeons should be formed to standardize the hospitals."[67] That it would also be a society that focused on surgical standardization was of less interest to Martin, who saw usefulness in a surgical focus only insofar as it might ultimately serve as a means of legitimate entry into the field of hospital standardization. The American College of Surgeons' surgical standardization program, Martin remarked to Codman, would serve as the "dog" that would "wag the tail" of hospital standardization. "The tail is more important than the dog," he announced his priorities to Codman, "but we shall have to have the dog to wag the tail."[68]

In Codman's retelling, then, the American College of Surgeons had to standardize surgery in order to gain the legitimacy and authority needed to achieve its real goal, which was the standardization of hospitals.[69] More than this, surgical standardization created an important impetus for hospital standardization. The requirements for surgical standardization, particularly the sharing of official records, laid bare the need for hospitals with standard recording practices. And even though the College cast its hospital standardization program as an organic next step, in Codman's telling it had been the goal from day one. Having convinced the surgical profession that it was the right standardizer of surgical practice, the College was, by 1919, ready to officially use its surgical standard dog to wag the tail of hospital standardization.

As Codman suggested, the College had already been planning this work for some time and, in fact, had secured $30,000 for it from the Carnegie Foundation back in 1916. Publicly, its shift in focus was predicated on promoting its surgical standardization program, citing hospital disorganization as the impediment to regulated surgical practice.[70] As Martin put it when recalling the College's efforts in standardization in 1923, the hospital standardization program was a by-product of surgeon accreditation. "We had to find a way of selecting our Fellows, and to judge . . . their ability as surgeons we had to know about their workshops and about the records of their workshops," he wrote.[71] The workshops of surgeons—the hospital—just happened to also be the workshops of medicine more generally.

To support this, the College declared that the fifty medical records plus fifty additional abstracts of surgical procedures required for fellowship were the most important pieces of evidence of surgical ability, without which a surgeon could not be admitted to membership. This was also the most difficult requirement to fulfill, since medical records, if they were kept at all, were typically kept at hospitals and not privately by surgeons themselves. Indeed, the College acknowledged that it initially had had to turn away 60 percent of prospective fellows because their case records were so fundamentally lacking.[72] Surgical standardization required, the College said, exactly that which most surgeons could not produce. And the problem lay with hospitals, where recordkeeping was hardly a standard feature. Although the value of medical records today is such a given that this step seems quite ordinary, before the College's required medical records for admission to its ranks, few hospitals kept them, and those that did were variable in what they recorded.[73]

Indeed, as Martin himself acknowledged in the 1930s, the grip the ACS had on standardization had been the culmination of a meticulously thought-out plan. That it succeeded, Martin suggested, was due to the fact that hospital standardization efforts had started "two or three years before [the medical community] realized what was going on," and so had had time to quietly percolate while the ACS built up its authority and legitimacy within medicine. "We finally convinced the surgeons that we were getting somewhere," he wrote, "and finally the whole medical profession realized the leadership in the American College of Surgeons."[74]

In both its early days and its recollection of them, the ACS made no mention of this strategy, instead repeating the messaging that sustained it through the initial criticisms of its surgical standardization program—that it was a democratic and meritocratic organization, serving the interests of society. Its standardization of surgery had simply brought a larger problem to light, and the ACS was the organization with the courage and the wherewithal to best tackle it. The ACS was an institution so filled with the "enthusiasm of youth and unhampered by tradition," as Martin put it, that it could "make itself responsible for the standardization of its own environment, the hospital."[75]

This rhetoric became increasingly important as the ACS began to sell its standardizing agenda to the general public. The Reverend Charles Moulinier, president of the Catholic Hospital Association and spokesperson for the ACS, waxed lyrical over the College's origins in a paper given at its 1921 hospital conference:

> The American College of Surgeons, stirred down into the depths of its soul, began to realize that it had a mission for the better care of the sick in the United States and Canada and made up its mind, as you all know and have been told, to improve surgery. But everybody also knows that you cannot improve surgery unless you improve everything that centers in the work of the hospital. And so the American College of Surgeons had not gone very far with its efforts and purpose to improve surgery when it realized that it had to improve everything in medicine.[76]

Of course, this "natural evolution" of the College's goals had been carefully cultivated.[77] Once fellowship in the ACS became a desired product, which it quite quickly did, it was but a short push to expand the College's work also to hospitals. What it needed now were standards that would ensure its broad applicability.

Unlike Flexner, who found in the Johns Hopkins Hospital the standard for his report on medical education, the ACS made a point of declaring that no hospital met its initial standard. Across the board, the College found, every medical institution was discovered to be shoddy, disorganized, and generally dysfunctional. Each hospital exhibited these qualities in incredibly variable ways, however, such that standard-setting at anything but the most minimal level could serve no purpose. Thus, the College cast itself as the only proper standard-bearer and established what it called its "minimum standard" by which hospitals would be judged. True to its name, there were very few requirements. Hospitals had to keep case records of their patients. The hospital and its staff were required to sign a morality pledge, chiefly confirming that the staff would not take part in the practice of fee-splitting.[78] The staff had to be organized and meet regularly, and the hospital needed to have a clinical laboratory.

This minimum standard was a new tactic for the ACS, one that aligned its work with those gurus of industrial efficiency, Gilbreth and Taylor, who held that purpose of a standard was a starting point rather than an end. As one of the College's fellows and spokespeople, Frederick Slobe, noted, the College's efforts in standardization were "not purported to be a resting place in the pathway" to progress. These initial efforts to achieve full conformity were only intended to produce a "safe foundation" from which "further advance," it was fervently hoped, would be "inevitable."[79]

Even so, the starting foundation was not large. Of the 692 hospitals surveyed in the first hospital standardization survey of 1919, only 89 were deemed to have met the minimum standard. The College made a point of saying that these 89 did *not* include some of the most well-known hospitals of the period, though it would not say precisely which hospitals had not passed. And, indeed, these are also lost to posterity, since the College, purportedly fearing that public release of the data would sow discord, decided to burn the results of this survey, sending up in flames the names of 89 institutions that had passed the standardizing test and the 603 that had failed it.[80] It was with this fiery flourish that the ACS announced the full-scale launch of its program.

Of course, a blanket declaration of condemnation and some charred remains was even more powerful than naming names. The hospital situation, as the College had surveyed it, was not just shoddy, it was *unspeakably, unreadably* shoddy. And its fair-minded, meritocratic approach to standardizing hospitals meant that every institution, even the major ones (or perhaps especially the major ones), had reason to worry about its status. Without having to release anything about its own methods or findings, the ACS had set itself up as the only and proper adjudicator of what a standard hospital should look like.

The hospital standardization effort of the College was not without its detractors, though by now the College had a strong foundation of legitimacy. Still, one strand of criticism persisted along familiar lines. Standardization of hospitals, went the naysayers, would lead not to further innovation but inevitably to dullness, sameness, and "mediocrity." As a spokesperson for the California League for the Conservation of Public Health explained, since "personality forms an essential and important part of the qualifications of the successful physician, so it must be for a hospital." This commentator continued:

> A hospital must have personality—a soul, if you please, and that personality must express itself constantly in idealism, service and efficiency. No two hospitals can be so alike, nor should they be alike—to make them so would lead to mediocrity. Each hospital has its own individual problems, and these problems must be solved by different remedies.[81]

In this invocation of a hospital's local conditions and environment, as well as in its emphasis on "personality," critics articulated a view that would only become more trenchant over time. It was a familiar concern from the industrial context—that standardization led to a general dulling and a loss of individuality because of its dehumanizing and deskilling logic. It was a trope that drove the satirical film *Modern Times*, in which the inimitable Charlie Chaplin literally loses himself to the autocratic standardizing logic of the assembly line by being incorporated bodily into the cogs of the factory machinery.[82]

Within medicine, though, the stakes were differently formulated. Rather than wring their hands at the loss of medical worker individuality, opponents of hospital standardization accused the project of posing a threat to patients, each of whom deserved the individualized care that standardization sought to drum out. Indeed, one of their go-to rebuttals to standardization was that medical treatment was effective precisely *because* it was not standard. They defined medical effectiveness, whether or not it actually halted disease entities, in terms of its local and individualized focus.[83] To them, medical efficacy would be weakened by standardization, since its power lay in treating individuals and communities, each in its own environment, rather than a universalized marketplace. In a refrain that is still familiar to us today, the push and pull of medical standardization began to turn on the perceived tension between personal medical care, which became increasingly prominent over this period, and the standardized medical care that in the preceding decades had been so necessary to medicine's modernization.

During the 1910s and 1920s, when the bulk of the College's programs took root, there were more proponents than opponents of standardization within medicine. In the College's marketing activities over the following two decades, however, the program of standardization came increasingly into tension with promises to protect or restore individualized care. Once again, the definition of medical effectiveness—and of what medicine's product would be—hung in the balance.

Standardization and the Black Hospitals

Among the many debates around standardization and the different values its methods might carry—from autocratic to democratic—it was always clear that these arguments, conversations, and decisions took place among the already enfranchised. Although the College's efforts to standardize may have included some marginal hospitals and surgeons that stood on the edges of the mainstream, it did not as a rule consider the state of Black hospitals or concern itself much with the status of Black surgeons and physicians. Black surgeons were not precluded from membership in the ACS, but apart from one surgeon who was automatically inducted based on his prestige, the College had only one other Black surgeon on its rolls before the 1940s.[84]

The egalitarianism and commitment to democracy and meritocracy that rhetorically framed the College's hospital standardization program clearly did not apply to the Black hospitals, whose more general disenfranchisement was manifested in the very circumstances of their formation. That is, white hospitals routinely excluded Black patients. Though some white hospitals in the North had adopted segregated wards, in the South, white hospitals were exclusively for white patients. As Vanessa Northington Gamble has put it, "The color line in hospital care was so rigid that even medical emergencies did not bend it."[85]

Partly for this reason, the Black hospitals that emerged in the South were not automatically inclined toward oversight. Though disenfranchisement came with multiple drawbacks, re-enfranchisement into a system like the College's meant—almost inevitably—closure, when it was found that they could not meet ACS standards. This helps to explain why a survey of the Black hospitals undertaken over the mid-1920s reported such a dismal response rate. Of 167 surveys sent out to known or suspected hospitals that served Black patients in 1927, only 57 responded.[86]

But there were other potential reasons for this dismal rate, explained H. M. Green, the president of the National Medical Association (NMA), the Black organization of physicians. Some Black hospitals were run by white, often religious organizations that did not identify themselves in terms of the patients they served and so thought their institutions outside the survey's scope. Some hospitals may have closed in the interim for lack of funds. And some preferred to remain uncounted, in part precisely so that their hospitals could retain their lack of oversight by public organizations. As he reported in 1928, either "from modesty or other reasons," some small hospitals "are unknown even to the postal officials of their own communities, and though reliably informed by their neighbors that they exist and are doing business, letters sent to them are returned marked 'Unclaimed.'"[87]

The worry that standardization might close Black hospitals outright or push them so far into financial precarity in the process of meeting these standards that they would not be able to survive was one founded on the experience of Flexner's study of medical education in 1910. In that case, only two Black medical schools were deemed fit enough to remain in operation. And although Flexner's report did not carry with it any sort of power to close hospitals on the spot, it influenced the funding decisions of the government and philanthropic organizations that kept medical schools open. This would only further jeopardize the health of twelve million Americans whose hospital options were already severely limited. As the physician Algernon Brashear Jackson put it in 1930, poor and few hospitals already spelled poorer health for Black patients than for white.[88] The further imposition of standards seemed far more likely to make matters worse than they were to bring the improvements in care that standardization purportedly promised.

Yet, the impact of standardization was not only read in terms of the direct impact it would have on the health of Black citizens.[89] Green laid it out for readers in the *Journal of the National Medical Association* in 1922, noting that also on the line was the possibility of Black Americans entering medicine as physicians or surgeons at all. Because of the close ties between standardized hospitals and accredited and standardized doctors—the very linkage the ACS exploited to get into hospital standardization in the first place—any further reduction of Black hospitals would mean a reduction in the training opportunities of Black physicians. Green noted that only 15 percent of Black hospitals in 1922 were large enough and had the capacity to train physicians, and these, he feared, might not meet even the College's minimal criteria. The remaining 85 percent, meanwhile, were a variable combination of small, makeshift, informal institutions that had neither training programs nor, in some cases, a visible footprint outside their own small communities.[90] If training opportunities disappeared for Black physicians, Green noted, it would be one more nail in the coffin of the already uphill battle to gain legitimacy and standing, not just for Black physicians but for Black professionals more broadly.

Green had reason to be worried. When Jackson undertook a survey of the Black hospitals in the United States in 1928 at the behest of the AMA, his observations painted a grim portrait. Although he didn't doubt that the "majority of our hospitals have been founded with the finest and highest intentions to render a most needed and helpful service," the reality, he wrote, was that they

> miss the mark all too often because of untrained and ignorant management, lack of professional co-operation, petty jealousies, poverty with its consequent poor equipment, lack of wholesome atmosphere within and without, and finally inadequate skill to do the job, bringing, as these menaces are bound to bring, public distrust, non-cooperation and loss of confidence which eventually spell failure.[91]

It was precisely to address these problems that members of the NMA founded the National Hospital Association (NHA) in 1923 to survey and then standardize the Black hospitals of the United States.[92] But while it succeeded in its advocacy for Black hospitals, as Gamble notes, it was not a successful revolution. Even if slightly more cooperation began to exist among the College, the AMA, the American Hospital Association, and the NHA around these issues, the end result was never an outpouring of funds to assist the Black hospitals in these tasks. And, indeed, most cooperative ventures began and ended at the survey stage.[93]

Part of the reason for the inability of the NHA to effectively solve the problem of the standardization of Black hospitals had to do with a longer-standing issue that standardization brought once more to the fore. For the NMA, the question of whether it should separately organize its own standardization program held no easy answer. If it did so, it risked condemnation by critics for being an agent of segregation. If it did not, it risked the survival of Black hospitals and, with that, the well-being of Black patients and training opportunities for Black medical professionals.[94]

This was not, of course, a dynamic of the NMA's own choosing. As Green put it, the worst part of the hospital standardization movement was not that there was a clear intention to put Black hospitals practitioners out of business, although it certainly would. Instead, it was that "they had not considered us at all." The impact of standardization on the Black medical institutions simply had not been taken into account. In a nod to the brand of institutional racism that ruled the day, even the minimal standard was focused on observed conditions at white hospitals exclusively, with the result that proposed standards and articulated interventions fit only these spaces.[95]

The situation was not dissimilar to that which had occasioned the founding of the NMA in 1895. In a move that neatly sidestepped any explicit policymaking on the issue of race, the AMA delegated decisions about membership to local societies, leaving Black physicians routinely excluded, especially in the

South. Though an artifact of the Reconstruction era, it was a policy that was left largely unchanged until the 1960s.[96]

Yet, of the estimated seven thousand doctors eligible for membership in 1922, the NMA had only about five hundred on its roll. This hamstrung the organization, limiting its funds, clout, and overall legitimacy.[97] And as Green crisscrossed the nation to drum up membership, it became clear that many were refusing to join because of the implicit support for a separate-and-unequal health care system that the NMA seemed to them to embody. This was particularly true in the North, where the majority of Black medical professionals lived and worked, having been drawn there, as Flexner would also discover, by the greater training and employment opportunities the region offered.

Still, the organizing efforts continued. As John Kenney, the editor of the *Journal of the National Medical Association*, put it in an editorial defending the NHA in 1926: "All too long some of us have hidden behind the fancied excuse of auto-segregation to justify our inactivity in regard to medical organizations and hospitals." But, he continued,

> We emphatically deny that by organizing our own medical societies and by establishing our own hospitals, we are segregating ourselves. As little as we like to place emphasis upon these things, we have to admit the color line is already drawn and that we are simply adapting ourselves to our environment, and if we do not meet the exigencies forced upon us by taking action along these lines, we are not meeting existing demands.[98]

In this, Kenney echoed the NMA's manifesto, penned in 1908 by founding member C. V. Roman. It stated that the organization had been "conceived in no spirit of racial exclusiveness, fostering no ethnic antagonism, but born of the exigencies of the American environment."[99]

To some observers, these organizational efforts had much in common with the Booker T. Washington school of thought.[100] That is, the Black hospital movement manifested a path toward cultural and political legitimacy through its demonstration of the ability of Black citizens to "solve their own problems, just like other segments of the society," as Gamble put it.[101] But the NHA did not ultimately signal the "Negro Hospital Renaissance" that Kenney, in 1930, had hoped for.[102] In part, as Flexner had already observed, this had to do with the fact that it was ultimately white philanthropies or government agencies that provided the funds—limited and prescriptive though they were—for the development of Black hospitals.[103] This went some of the way toward shoring up some of the larger hospitals, and maintaining the opportunity for training, but it also meant that the smaller, more informal hospitals that had arisen out of the sheer absence of local care were left to fend for themselves. Many of these were put out of business by the Depression. Some did not even survive this long.[104] The result was a handful of successful hospitals, surrounded by a sea of institutions struggling to survive.

But it was also clear that white charity was not an optimal, or perhaps even a viable, path toward racial integration. And it was this view that prevailed after World War II, when the small inroads the NMA and NHA had made in shoring up the Black hospitals were tallied up and found extremely wanting. This time, though, the NMA did not have a goal of adding hospitals to what was now described as a "poorly financed black medical ghetto." Instead, it joined the National Association for the Advancement of Colored People (NAACP) in arguing that a segregated health care system was unacceptable and inequitable in every conceivable way—including in terms of health outcomes.[105]

Perhaps the efforts of the NMA and the NHA did manage to help Black medical practitioners retain a place in medical training and a stake, however small, in the larger public debate about health care.[106] There are certainly other stories to join Gamble's in telling about the Black hospital movement over the larger sweep of the twentieth century. Here, though, their struggles reveal a darker significance for standardization. For Black medical practitioners and institutions of the era, it represented neither innovation nor democracy nor populism. The product of modern medicine was social, political, and economic exclusion.

4

The Labor

Over-production is stamped on the face of these facts.—THE FLEXNER REPORT, 1910

In 1890, the education reformer Abraham Flexner founded a school in his hometown of Louisville, Kentucky. Its name, Mr. Flexner's School, was quite a bit less radical than its pedagogical premise: to offer a reformist alternative to the well-entrenched curricular conventions of the day by dispensing completely with lectures, exams, and grades in favor of small, lively group discussions. Flexner's educational experiment was considered a success—one that many educators across the country would later attempt to reproduce. When he collected his thoughts on the subject in a pamphlet titled *A Modern School*, however, the reformer cautioned that his model should not be replicated: successful and truly educational institutions functioned best, he wrote, when each paid attention to the specific needs of its pupils and drew on local assets—its "accessible world"—in crafting a curriculum.[1] In essence, effective education could not be standardized. To those who know his name today, it is perhaps surprising that Flexner would hold these beliefs. After all, he was soon to become the figurehead of a national standardization campaign credited with the systematic removal of variation from the landscape of medical education.[2]

Flexner eventually sold his school for a profit, and in 1908, he published a book on higher education titled *The American College*. It did not sell well. That same year, Flexner found himself in New York City in search of employment. Among his appointments was a visit with Henry Pritchett, a like-minded education critic and the president of Andrew Carnegie's educationally focused philanthropic endeavor, the Carnegie Foundation for the Advancement of Teaching. The two apparently hit it off, and Pritchett, appreciating Flexner's reformist flair, offered the educator a job: the evaluation of the 155 medical schools of the United States and Canada.[3] Worried that Pritchett might have confused him with his better-known physician brother Simon, Flexner initially balked. After all, he knew nothing about medical education. But Pritchett insisted that he had the right Flexner, and Abraham relented, setting himself to the task that would make his name far more medically memorable than his brother's.

It took just two years for Flexner to complete his survey of medical education. In 1910, he published the report of his efforts, which appeared as *Carnegie Bulletin Number 4*, under the title "Medical Education in the United States and Canada: A Report to the Carnegie Foundation for the Advancement of Teaching." The work was so quickly and strongly associated with Flexner himself, though, that in short time it became known as "Mr. Flexner's Report" and later, the "Flexner Report." By the midpoint of the year, fifteen thousand copies of the heavily promoted and widely disseminated publication had been sent out into the world, arriving to most recipients for the cost of postage alone.[4] Excerpts of the document were seeded in the popular press, and local and national news outlets ran story after story about the study's remarkable—and shocking—findings. Pritchett wanted everybody to read it. By year's end, it was difficult to find a corner of the United States that had not at least heard of Flexner and the Carnegie Foundation.

The Flexner Report, like Flexner himself, has had a tumultuous afterlife. In medical circles, it has been celebrated as a fundamentally transformative document that shaped the successful regime of medical education and catapulted American medical practice to international renown.[5] For Flexner's contemporaries, the report was not itself *the* revolution but instead a critical "catalyst" of a generally salutary systematization of medicine that was already taking place.[6]

Over the 1970s and 1980s, the report went from fame to infamy. It was a moment when many actions of the American Medical Association (AMA) across the previous half century were being reassessed and newly critiqued, and Flexner's work was found guilty by association. Because it had been at least inspired if not explicitly commissioned by the AMA, the report was held up as evidence of the AMA's ruthless efforts to consolidate and control the medical profession and its complicity with large-scale philanthropy in turning medicine into a thoroughly capitalist and corrupted enterprise.[7]

Indeed, though his work at the time was not very different from that of the American College of Surgeons, it was Flexner who came to be associated with a vaguely construed but deeply intuited notion of medical capitalism. In so many ways, he is an easy target. His advocacy for streamlining medical education that would keep only the *best* medical schools—judged to be so mainly by their similarity to his favored model, Johns Hopkins—certainly smacks of elitism, ensuring that medicine remained an exclusive club of mostly white men who were at the very least middle class.

Then there was his follow-up work: vigorously supporting his chosen programs with the enormous infusions of cash that he was privy to at the Carnegie Foundation and then the Rockefeller Foundation—organizations, critics said, created in large part to rehabilitate the tarnished reputations of their monopolistic patrons. That these philanthropic foundations had extensive ties to the AMA was not immaterial. As the socially minded historians of the 1970s saw it, it was a story of collusion that produced the structure of medical economics and power that remain our inheritance.[8]

But although the Flexner Report's legacy is certainly the elitist, exclusionist medical educational system we have today, Flexner considered his standardization work to be something far different from an exercise in the capitalist logic of control. His work may have acquired a level of infamy far and above that of other standardizing outfits operating in the same period, but it was Flexner who, more eloquently and loudly than most, expressed the conflicts inherent in standardization.[9]

Indeed, even as he advocated for standardizing and streamlining medical education, the reduction of medical schools, and the more efficient distribution of medical practitioners across the country in his famous report, Flexner had other reforms on his mind. In his writings, he critiqued the dull, homogenous, and ineffective training that students encountered first in the secondary schools and then in the colleges; he advocated for the "democratic" (as opposed to the "aristocratic" model of the "Old World") mode of education that he saw as unique to, and uniquely possible in, the United States; and he called for the instillation of democracy-adjacent qualities like "freedom" and "liberty" in education, even if, like others, he struggled mightily with questions about how these qualities ought to be manifested and how standardizers could create and maintain the delicate balance between meaningful standards, on the one hand, and meaningful flexibility and creativity within a static educational curriculum, on the other.[10]

This tension between Flexner the medical standardizer and Flexner the educational reformer comes out in his later writings. In a 1925 book on medical education, for example, he laments the negative impacts of his work on standardizing medical education.[11] Flexner's reforms did take on a life of their own over time, and the mores of medical education that became the norm in the United States—which are, at their worst, nightmarishly elitist, exclusive, and rigid—were probably not what Flexner had in mind. But this does not mean that Flexner was an *unwitting* participant in the standardization of medical education.

Instead, it may be useful to think of the Flexner Report and its legacy as a salient example of what Louis Brandeis, the trustbuster and Supreme Court justice, considered the problem of "bigness." That is, though many large organizations were able to grow large by means of efficiency, once they reached a certain size, efficiency would no longer be sustainable. At that point, their very bigness fostered a sort of harmful *inefficiency*, by which Brandeis meant graft, greed, and reprehensibly monopolistic behavior.[12] If it did not succumb to inefficiency on its own, Brandeis suggested, it would surely not be allowed to survive by others in the marketplace who could not compete with it. By way of example, he pointed to Andrew Carnegie's US Steel, which had acquired its size by efficiency methods of which Brandeis approved but had been bought out by a duplicitous steel trust precisely because it had become *too* efficient.[13]

Though Brandeis's view has been subsequently regarded as too reductive, it marks at least one contemporary strand of reformist thought: standardization and efficiency had a maximum size or space of application, beyond which it would start to decay into something else—a handmaiden of monopoly, perhaps. Though in much more complex terms, this is arguably the crucial difference between the application of Henry Ford's business philosophy to his own businesses and the global Fordism that shot an iteration of American capitalism around the world. Though a mixed bag of ideological commitments at the local factory level, it became a dominant, oppressive force for capitalism when it exceeded those limits.[14]

Without taking Brandeis's potentially pathologic distaste for bigness too far, this chapter thus takes the Flexner Report as a kind of efficiency boundary object—one that sits uncomfortably between efficiency and its local application within medicine, on one side, and the "bigness" of capitalism and power, on the other. It is a useful way of thinking about this work, in no small part because it also catapulted the problems of medicine into the mainstream by drawing direct parallels with other problematic manifestations of cultural, political, and economic crisis.

Though much of the chapter is concerned with charting this transformation, it ends with what was in many ways the clearest sign that the standardization of medical education had become fully rendered in capitalist terms. In deciding who gets left out of medical education, the end result of the Flexner Report would be a legacy of political exclusion.[15]

The Report

Historically, the significance of the Flexner Report has turned a great deal on how one reads the intentions of the actors involved. The point of contention seems to be chiefly this: although the Carnegie Foundation headlined the report, it was actually proposed—or by some accounts, covertly commissioned— by Arthur Dean Bevan, the head of the Council on Medical Education at the AMA.[16] In 1907, Bevan had approached Pritchett with the idea that the Carnegie Foundation might continue and extend the work that the AMA had already begun: the in-person evaluation of every medical school in the United States and Canada. Critical to this task was the appointment of a nonmedical and thus apparently unbiased evaluator (Flexner) who would conduct the study alongside the AMA's own in-house medical school evaluator, N. P. Colwell.[17]

Older accounts tend to suggest that the rationale for this move, on the part of the AMA, was to turn over this evaluative role to an objective arbiter who, minus the entangling alliances and political niceties that forced the AMA to hold its tongue on the educational status of certain institutions, could say with greater candor and precision what the state of medical education really looked like.[18]

Later historians, however, simply saw an ill-concealed complicity between the AMA and the Carnegie Foundation—a shared desire to control medical education, with benefits for both. The Foundation would boost its profile as a civic-minded agent of social reform while the AMA would bring a diverse and unruly population of medical practitioners into line under its control.

However one reads the significance of the report, the drama and flair that Flexner imparted to it is beyond debate. Across its pages, Flexner exercised his impressive vocabulary of disdain at the expense of a wide range of medical institutions. The press loved it, and quotes from the Flexner Report appeared in articles across the United States and Canada. The report's findings were also enthusiastically amplified by Pritchett himself, in outlets ranging from local newspapers to prominent national journals.[19]

An article in the business-centric *World's Work* showcased some of Flexner's best put-downs. He called one of the worst medical colleges he visited—the California Medical College in Los Angeles—"a disgrace to the state." Then there was the Georgia College of Eclectic Medicine and Surgery in Atlanta, of which Flexner wrote, "Nothing more disgraceful calling itself a medical school can be found anywhere." This, seemingly, was before he visited the medical schools of Chicago. Apparently feeling that the critique of any single school could not suffice to show the depths of his pedagogical despair, he wrote that the whole city should be considered "the plague spot of the country" when it came to medical education.[20]

Flexner also expressed his horror at discovering that medical schools opening in the autumn would often graduate their first "doctors" the following spring, so as to make sure that their reputation was associated with success in the production of diplomaed doctors from the very start.[21] Because licensing requirements had been sacrificed on the altar of Jacksonian democracy in the early nineteenth century and only very recently reappeared, they were generally minimal and quite variable. As a result, a diploma remained almost by itself a license to practice medicine in 1910. These newly minted doctors could begin their work immediately, mixing in and becoming almost undetectable—Flexner ominously pointed out to his readers—from their better-educated peers.[22]

Though Flexner had barbs to spare, the primary targets of the report were the commercial or "proprietary schools" that owed their existence to the profit motives of the groups of physicians who opened them. This was a model that turned a profit when costs were kept low and student populations high. As a result, Flexner noted, the physical state of these schools was dreadful, with most comprised of a "cheaply rented" hall, "rude benches," and occasionally a "skeleton—in whole or in part—and a box of odd bones."[23] But while these schools skimped on supplies, they spent extravagantly on marketing. "They may be uncertain about the relation of the clinical laboratory to bedside instruction," Flexner noted derisively, "but they have calculated to a nicety which 'medium' brings the largest 'return.'"[24]

For these revelations, Flexner chose a particular historical backdrop. Like many reforming practitioners, Flexner waxed nostalgic about the eighteenth-century model of medicine, idealized as a moment in which medical education was reserved for those who could afford the leisurely overseas sojourn to tour the preeminent medical institutions of Europe that it generally entailed.[25] It was the nineteenth century that lay at the heart of the problem—the same tendency toward populism that had turned education into what he considered a hopeless variety show had done the same to medicine. The medical sects that proliferated in that period had set up their own educational institutions, each with its own set of standards.

Flexner specifically dated the crisis he saw in front of him to the early nineteenth-century opening of a single medical school in Maryland: the "so-called medical department," he scoffed, "of the so-called University of Maryland."[26] According to Flexner, that proprietary school established the unhealthy precedent from which every other proprietary school took inspiration. Its lack of an affiliation to a real university, which Flexner believed grounded professional schools pedagogically and introduced a necessary system of educational standards, meant that it was an educational institution completely unmoored and unregulated. It was not a "branch growing out of the living university trunk," as Flexner put it, but rather an impostor, disconnected from the "standards and ideals" of the proper university and out for only one thing: profits. The independent, proprietary medical schools that followed in its footsteps would be the "fertile source of unforeseen harm to medical education and to medical practice."[27]

The proprietary school model proliferated, growing steadily during the nineteenth century. "Between 1810 and 1840, twenty-six new medical schools sprang up," Flexner noted. "Between 1840 and 1876, forty-seven more; the number actually surviving in 1876 ha[d] since then much more than doubled." Indeed, a whopping 457 new medical schools had been created since 1810. Many were "short-lived" and "perhaps fifty still-born," Flexner noted.[28] But the investment required was so minimal that once a school closed, perhaps having exhausted the market for medical diplomas for a time in one area, another might shortly thereafter open, remaining in place until it too had taken all the fees it could.

The most lucrative aspect of the schools, Flexner continued, was in many instances not the fees accrued from students but the relationships—the fiduciary networks—created among students and their teachers. After students finished their education, they often referred their patients back to their instructors because they had no idea what to do themselves. According to an "old joke" in medical education, the first thing these hapless proprietary school–educated practitioners did when encountering a patient, even in an emergency, was to call for a consultation with their erstwhile professors.[29]

These consultations from their underqualified but loyal former students became an additional, reliable profit stream for medical school instructors. Among other things, it was a situation that made clear to Flexner that the priorities of these medical schools lay not in being educational institutions but in presenting profitable and extremely self-serving networking opportunities. Indeed, so lucrative could medical education be in this regard that there were reports of physicians paying dearly for chairs at these institutions because of the lifelong consultation fees that would invariably follow.[30]

Though the great majority of Flexner's lyrical tirades were reserved for these proprietary institutions, he noted that the nineteenth-century poisoning of medical education had reached even the prominent old universities. Flexner singled out Harvard, Yale, and the University of Pennsylvania as key examples of venerable institutions whose medical schools had succumbed to the proprietary school spirit. Though these schools had nominally retained their relationship to their universities, the "wave of commercial exploitation which swept the entire profession" led to the same behavior that one saw at the less reputable schools. They operated independently from their universities and collected fees that were divided exclusively among the medical faculty. Professorships were decided by vote so that popularity rather than skill was rewarded. And students were hustled through to graduation in the same diploma mill fashion, prioritizing popularity, family connections, and other intangibles over and above ability.[31] At Harvard, as long as a majority of the nine-professor graduating committee voted for any student to graduate, they received their diploma.[32]

It was really only Johns Hopkins University, a youthful thirty-four years old in 1910, that was spared Flexner's disdain. Indeed, Hopkins, Flexner's own alma mater, and its medical school, where his brother Simon had completed his postgraduate training, were the "one bright spot" on the otherwise desolate landscape of medical education. In Baltimore was a medical school that he rather melodramatically described as "small but ideal . . . embodying in a novel way, adapted to American conditions, the best features of medical education in England, France and Germany." The school became Flexner's model institution, the one against which all other institutions would be measured and from which the right standard of medical education would emerge.[33]

Though other commentators would later infer it, Flexner's Report stays largely silent on the connection between poorly trained practitioners and patient health.[34] In fact, the through line between educational quality and practitioner ability that we now take for granted was not self-evident at the time. In part, this was because, although there were curative breakthroughs, especially at the turn of the twentieth century (the development of the dramatically lifesaving diphtheria antitoxin is a commonly cited example), in this moment of incredible enthusiasm for efficiency, the "science" of medicine from which we now impute much of medicine's significance was rendered in other terms.[35] As Flexner explained in 1925:

There is a widespread impression that the scientific quality of medical education and medical practice is in some fashion dependent upon the part played by the laboratory. This is not the case. Science is essentially a matter of observation, inference, verification, generalization. The mind of [Thomas] Sydenham, interested in a sick child and humanely preoccupied with its cure, did not, in so far as it functioned scientifically, operate differently from that of Galileo, interested in cosmic physicians. Both alike observed, reflected, verified, generalized.[36]

For Flexner, as for others working in this same reformist vein, medical efficacy was achieved primarily through organization over and above nearly everything else. To them, only efficiency interventions like standardization and record-keeping would yield the transformation that medicine needed.

In part, this reflected the disorganized everyday reality of medicine on the ground. The plurality of medical "sects" that had emerged from the nineteenth-century waves of populism meant that practitioners of homeopathy, allopathy (what we now consider mainstream medicine), osteopathy, chiropractic, eclecticism, and other forms of medical practice dotted the country, each with their own training schools, and each believing their views on medicine and its effective practice to be the best, with none really able to prove definitively the superiority of their practices over any other. And in every sect, including the "regulars," as the allopathic medical practitioners called themselves, there were fraudulent, disreputable practitioners.[37] Despite the diversity of medical imaginaries, the chaotic nature of the medical world in which practitioners operated made reform one of their few common goals. Plans for the different sects to collaborate in reform efforts—for example, by setting up medical schools that could offer a standardized curriculum that amalgamated the best practices from each medical sect—were circulated relatively widely.[38]

And indeed, the point of the medical education horror story that the Flexner Report told to the public was not that the haplessness of poorly educated practitioners might cause the death of their loved one or themselves in some sort of direct doctor-patient encounter gone wrong. Where patients were a consideration for Flexner, it came in terms of patients in aggregate, in which case medicine ballooned as a category to include "preventive medicine, sanitation and public health" and effectiveness evaluated by the general efficiency and productivity of the population. Where patients as individuals are mentioned in the report, it is not in terms of their potentially untimely demise or continued disability as much as it is the travesty of the unstandardized care they might receive.[39] "That sick man," Flexner disapprovingly noted, "is relatively rare for whom actually all is done that is at this day humanly feasible." This variability of product reflected the troubling variability and corruption of the medical practitioner population. "There is probably no other country in the world," he despaired, "in which there is so great a distance and so fatal a difference between the best, the average, and the worst."[40]

In this way, the Flexner Report was less about the mores of medicine as we understand them today and much more about a mode and definition of medical effectiveness that rested on the prevailing logic of modernization. The scandal was not that medicine was ineffective or that people were dying as a result of the persistence of these proprietary institutions. It was that these proprietary institutions were disorganized and antidemocratic, at a moment when these were cardinal cultural sins.

For Flexner, the problem was a familiar one, and its possible solutions were quite thorny. As an educational reformer, he had applauded to some degree the same populist spirit that had given rise to the capitalist and commercialist proprietary forms of medical education. It was a push for universal education that rejected the stale old educational forms that had been brought over with the colonists, the primary purpose of which, he said, had been "to secure the type; to renew and fortify the old English Puritan" and to produce the "detached and learned class" that typified the aristocratic, antidemocratic European societies from that of the United States.[41]

What Flexner explicitly wanted to avoid replicating in the United States was the role of education as a means "to maintain the present social organization stable and intact. . . . The more thorough they are educationally, the more effectual they are as a means of social constraint."[42] By contrast, in the democracy that was the United States, "society" was always "regarded as in process of making," and thus education "must first of all prepare [students] to participate in activities which it is open to [them] also to modify by the creative outcome of [their] own endeavors."[43] In a country defined by "social plasticity" rather than "social constraint," the role of education was to raise each individual up: to create citizens who were equipped to govern, since this is what a democracy called on its people to do.[44]

Education done well, then, would allow for the kind of overcoming of classism and social constraint that so limited European society. But that had yet to happen. Instead, a kind of populism within educational institutions had resulted in few if any standards at all, leading to a situation where education could not fulfill the crucial function of imparting social plasticity and democratic values. Echoing a familiar angst over standardization, Flexner wrote that "we are forbidden to adjust the college to existing social conditions through definite organization" because to do so required a homogenization or attrition of some of the competing educational values that proponents of these values would not allow.[45] Where standardization was guided by populism, there was no hope of stability, consistency, or quality in standards. The result was just a superabundance of choices. "Pending the elucidation of the problem of values," Flexner wrote, "no particular values are respected. There is no agreement as to what is more, what less important; as to what is essential, and what incidental or instrumental" within education.[46]

The result was a mess: schools didn't teach, students didn't learn, and the production of the capable, democratic individuals a democratic society demanded was not taking place. It was an essentially undemocratic and "thoroughly immoral" situation. Flexner concluded that "[the college's] demoralization of standards simply expresses the fact that, as it serves no particular educational purpose, it is immaterial whether the student takes the thing seriously or not."[47]

Thus, Flexner signaled his allegiance to the reformist standardization principles of the day. These were also the tenets that guided the Carnegie Foundation, as Pritchett himself made clear when writing in defense of the Foundation in 1915. Its interests as a "standardizing agency" were not in the "mechanical standardization" of universities by dint of arbitrary imposition. Instead, the Foundation followed the standard efficiency procedure: first, to explicate current standards so that they could be interrogated, discussed, and through this process, agreed on. Only then could decisions be made about a step-wise system to improve standards. And on this note, Pritchett said, what was needed was not more independence on the part of each university to decide what their standards would be. That had only led down the path to an elective system that, like the mania for invention that the editors of the *Modern Hospital* observed in their own attempts to standardize, only produced chaos. Instead, what was required was a system-wide discussion of standard-setting in the name of a notion of educational "freedom": a term defined here as the full functioning of the university as a democratic institution for the good of the people.[48] Echoing in this way the view that standards were not an end in themselves but rather a waypoint to the establishment of an ideal, both Pritchett and Flexner understood standards as technical tools instead of absolute goals. Still, using standardization to achieve a democratic ideal was a difficult needle to thread.[49] Flexner attempted to do exactly that with his report, using medical education as an experimental space to test an array of powerful standardizing tools.

The Method

The Flexner Report captured the public's attention and directed it to the problematic state of medical education, an achievement that Flexner accomplished largely by dramatically framing the issue as part of a wider cultural story. Though the report was clearly a statement about medical education with explicit ramifications about how modern medicine would develop, it was simultaneously an exposé of the existence and persistence of a phenomenon that seemed to be popping up everywhere in twentieth-century American life: unstandardized, unrationalized, and essentially corrupt institutions that embodied the worst of what we would now call capitalist tendencies. It probably made for fascinating but familiar reading to the American public. Flexner was not just a reformer—he was a muckraker.

Indeed, the Flexner Report can be read as but the latest chapter in a journalistic tradition that had started in the nineteenth century. Among muckraking's first targets, then, had been "bossism," exemplified by the infamous Boss Tweed of New York's most powerful political machine, Tammany Hall.[50] From there, the tradition went to explore more widely the corrupting influence of money and large businesses. As the famous muckraker Lincoln Steffens wrote in one of his turn-of-the-century exposés of local government, "Politics is business—that's what's the matter with it. That's what's the matter with everything—art, literature, religion, journalism, law, medicine—they're all business."[51]

And from the start, the Flexner Report was all business. In his introduction to the report, Pritchett painted proprietary schools as akin to trusts—those same corporate entities that Brandeis had excoriated as operating extra-efficiently, and thus also deviously and illegally, to shore up their power. This would be a familiar theme throughout the report: the poisonous and damaging actions of a dangerously unlimited Goliath—in this case, the ephemeral but no less nefarious proprietary medical schools that had insinuated themselves even into the venerable old universities—versus the "small but ideal" David, here cast as the youthful Johns Hopkins.[52] The instability wrought by the large corporate entities—the greed, graft, and thoroughly antidemocratic behavior that the muckrakers exposed as the backbone of these corporate machines—had a clear medical analogue in the money-grubbing practices of the proprietary, for-profit medical schools.[53] In terms of social, economic, and political stability, medicine was just as urgently in need of reform as those industries already exposed as broken and exploitative—meatpacking, oil, steel, tobacco, and corrupted government itself.

Business was not the only theme, however. Another narrative in the Flexner Report was the concept of overproduction, a problem that the AMA had made much of in its earlier standardizing efforts. As one medical commentator had put it in 1901, the same "principles of political economy" that applied to the "output of a machine shop" applied equally to medicine. But unlike the product of a machine shop, which, he suggested, could be sold abroad, doctors were a domestic product only. Minus the "recourse of foreign markets" that manufacturers enjoyed, he explained, the overproduction of doctors resulted in a dire situation indeed.[54] The glut of physicians was wreaking havoc on the medical marketplace.[55]

A decade down the road, overproduction would become famous as the answer to a burning question about the Great Depression: How had the boom of mass production resulted in the bust of the Depression's dramatic economic downturn? By the time of the Flexner Report, overproduction had already been marked out as a potential threat to economic, political, and cultural stability. It made sense, for with this era of mass production came not only enthusiasm for the efficiency that had created it but anxiety over what this newfound supply, sometimes surfeit, of stuff might bring.[56]

Thus, Flexner moved adeptly from a story of corruption to an efficiency analysis of the superabundance that the proliferation of "doctor-factories" was producing.[57] Shifting the emphasis from the greed and graft of the proprietary school operators, he described a more systemic crisis of medical education in terms of the imbalance that overproduction had created. Rather than rooting out corrupted practitioners, which might have been the answer had Flexner left his analogizing just to the muckrakers, Flexner advised gaining control of the whole of medical practice by streamlining it at its point of production: effectively turning it into a powerful rationalizing machine that would also rationalize the market more generally.

In his report, Flexner set production as the relevant aspect of the proprietary school problem early on by reciting a set of statistics that had been making the rounds in the medical literature. In Germany, he said, the ratio of physician to population was somewhere in the range of 1 per 2,000 in general, with about 1 in 1,000 in large cities. This was already judged to be a bit on the high side. But it was nothing as compared to the United States, where there was "1 doctor for every 568 persons." In large cities, Flexner noted, switching metrics, there was "frequently one doctor for every 400^2 [sic] or less." And in some small towns, Flexner exclaimed, residents sometimes could end up with "two or three physicians apiece!"[58]

Flexner's concern extended also to the distribution of physicians, which the surplus physicians produced by the proprietary schools had failed to ameliorate. "It is clear that even long-continued over-production of cheaply made doctors cannot force distribution beyond a certain well-marked point," he noted.⁵⁹ Doctors were not filling medical vacuums across the country. Instead, they were congregating in the cities and in wealthy towns with the goal of earning a good living. The result was fierce competition among physicians, with few receiving a steady income.

Reports of the uncertain finances of medical practitioners had indeed flooded the medical news in the decade before the Flexner Report. One doctor dramatically illustrated his story of how bad things had gotten by describing his encounter with a colleague who was "crying because he was hungry."⁶⁰ The average salary of a physician had certainly fallen, so that it was now less than that of a "telegraph operator working in an important office," as one writer put it with peculiar specificity. Neither telegraph operators of important offices nor physicians were falling into abject poverty, but neither could easily afford to buy and maintain a car, as an article in the *Journal of the American Medical Association* noted in driving home just how low the social and economic fortunes of the medical practitioners had fallen.⁶¹

But these weren't Flexner's stakes.⁶² Instead, his report was preoccupied with a concern for the social imbalance that the unacceptable problem of overproduction connoted. To a generation of Americans culturally primed to shun inefficiency, Flexner's description of doctor-factory overproduction as "something worse than waste" was meaningful indeed. His rationale for reform rested not on the personal crises of income experienced by some doctors but on the variability, instability, and inequitable and therefore antidemocratic populism that had been introduced into the market by too many unstandardized medical schools. The schools did a disservice to their students by virtue of their populist ethos, and then they destabilized the market by creating a wide range of doctors of such variable training and ability that their diplomas were largely meaningless. They were not "educated" per se, just as those who attended the totally unstandardized colleges were not educated. Nothing had been gained in this process except the profiting of corrupted institutions. In this sense, it was less any explicit belief in the rightness of allopathic medicine particularly that drove Flexner, although there is little doubt he was an adherent. It was more that the complete absence of standards resulted in exactly what Flexner had been trying to drive out of education more broadly.

Flexner noted repeatedly in his educational manifestos that the problems he saw in education had already been solved in other areas of economic life, where standards had been imposed for the sake of producing a functional democracy.⁶³ So it was probably not difficult for him to conjure up another analogue to clarify to his audience the problem of medical overproduction.

He did this in his report notably in terms set by the contemporary concept of Gresham's law.

Coined in 1860, Gresham's law was on the minds of turn-of-the-century Americans, thanks in part to William Jennings Bryan's ostentatious support of "bimetallism"—the "free silver" movement—as a plank in his currency reform platform. Bryan's opponents relied on Gresham's law for their arguments for maintaining the gold standard. It suggested that when the commodity values of the coins in a currency differed—as they would in Bryan's bimetallic proposition—whatever the face value of the coin, those coins with the higher commodity value would disappear from common use. After all, who would use a gold coin when a less valuable silver one of the same denomination would suffice to pay the same debts? The smelting of gold into bullion would almost certainly begin, as would its hoarding, and therefore withdrawal, from circulation. For this reason, as the "Gold Democrat" William Dallas Bynum put it in 1896, "Two kinds of money of unequal value cannot circulate side by side in the same country. The cheaper will always drive out the dearer."[64]

This was precisely the case in medical education, argued Flexner. The problematic variability of medical labor was not just damaging on its face—it would also prove unsustainable, following the natural order of things as dictated by Gresham's law. Low-grade material—whether of the proprietary medical school educated type, the medical sects, or just the more general dregs of the medical profession—would ultimately, inevitably float to the surface if variability were allowed to guide medicine. For these reasons, Flexner pressed home his point that unstandardized, unregulated medicine was guaranteed not only to be destabilizing but also ineffective and inequitable.

Without requiring Flexner to take sides in particular, his use of Gresham's law helped support the notion that the streamlining of medical practitioner production, rather than reform that would root out corruption but keep the variability of practitioners intact, had to take place as a matter of urgency. To be sure, a standard product was no guarantor of high quality. But with its power to remove variability, it was a crucial safeguard against low quality and its attendant dangers.

The Poor Boy

There were many critiques of the Flexner Report, especially from those who found themselves on the wrong side of the standardization that his evaluation suggested. For some, both in his own time and later, the fact that Flexner's work looked a lot like the AMA's suggested that he was merely an instrument of what would come ominously to be called "organized medicine." And indeed, it was true. The report did a great deal to shore up the particular aims and goals of the AMA, spelled out in terms of driving out "irregular" physicians, stabilizing the income of allopathic practitioners, and buoying medicine's sinking socioeconomic status.[65]

It is not surprising, then, that one common and biting strand of criticism was that the AMA was actually the real medical trust, rather than the proprietary medical schools that Pritchett had gone after.[66] As one writer deployed the term, the activities of this "medical trust" were even more egregious than those industrial trusts it was accused of emulating: it was like "Standard Oil Company go[ing] to the legislature," as one commentator put it, "to have statutes enacted saying 'No one can sell oil except our company.'"[67]

But, by far, one of the most popular talking points for critics of the Flexner Report was its premise that the standardization of medical education would ultimately lead away from autocratic, elitist, and rigid structures, to the egalitarian democracy that standardization more broadly promised. The case was notably made through what became known as the "poor boy" argument, which suggested that rather than advantage individuals from poorer, more rural areas by giving them an educational system that would be actually transformative, the standardization of medical education would instead cut off any medical opportunity for them altogether. And not only that, the absence of these medical practitioners would severely impact those areas that they had served—often, the selfsame poor, rural areas they had come from. Many places would likely now find themselves without any medical practitioners at all.

This had been one of the defenses that proprietary schools had drawn on in arguing for their continued existence: however deficient their curriculum, they nevertheless offered crucial educational opportunity to those who could not afford the hefty fees of the more elite universities, in places where medical practitioners would not otherwise distribute themselves. Flexner dismissed this logic, saying that it simply played on public sympathies in order to draw attention away from the malfeasances of the "poor school."[68]

But critics found ready ammunition for their poor boy argument in the Flexner family archive, latching onto the fact that it was the Flexner family's poverty that had led Flexner's older brother Simon to go to medical school at the decidedly unstoried, uncelebrated University of Louisville Medical Department.[69] This was the same institution, they noted gleefully, that Flexner had so recently derided in his report as "a popular medical center for crude boys thronged from the plantations" with "unmanageably huge" classes, "overcrowded" laboratories, and "meager" clinical facilities.[70]

That Simon Flexner had become the first director of the Rockefeller Institute for Medical Research after coming from a school for "crude boys" made for an excellent talking point among the report's detractors. Surely, the fact that the elder Flexner had attended this supposedly abysmal institution and yet had become one of the country's medical leaders should mean something. At the least, it pointed out that the uniform condemnation of medical education as corrupt was flawed—whether or not the University of Louisville had shortchanged him on his medical education, Simon had clearly flourished after his time there. Not only had this school made his career possible, but his attendance proved that there were future medical luminaries at even the poorest institutions of medical education.

It was a good argument against what critics perceived to be a larger agenda of defining and controlling the shape of medical labor along lines that privileged the wealthy and punished the poor.[71] As they saw it, Flexner's Report was an obvious attempt to establish certain norms for a new medical laboring class by delimiting from the outset who could and could not gain access to it. Indeed, all medical colleges for women, then, and all but two of the Black medical colleges were criticized in Flexner's report. These were judgments he touted as being rationalized on the basis of merit and determined by the "objective" study of these colleges.

It was Pritchett, and not Flexner, who responded to claims that Flexner's report would have put his own exceptional brother out of medicine. Simon Flexner's training at the University of Louisville, he announced, had actually amounted to very little. Only after being discovered by none other than William Welch, the celebrated head of the Johns Hopkins Medical School, had Simon Flexner's education begun. Pritchett bemoaned the fact that the older Flexner brother had to go to the low-quality Louisville institution, opining that if such schools did not exist, he would have instead attended a higher-quality college and thus achieved still greater medical fame.[72] Pritchett's sober but ludicrous spin was that Simon Flexner's storied career should actually be viewed as a great loss: the loss of a career that might have been even more storied had only the medical education system been fixed so that he could have attended a better institution.

Perhaps Flexner did not consider these family attacks worthy of a reply, but he certainly had one: by his logic, his brother Simon was exemplary of those deserving poor boys who would rise to the top regardless of their circumstance. The question for him wasn't really what Simon would have missed out on had these proprietary schools not been in place, but rather, what he would have gained had the rational system of education that Flexner set forth already been adopted. Either way, to Flexner, the motivated and talented "poor boy" would always achieve his destiny.[73]

In the end, the critics were proved right. The high-minded reforms envisioned by Flexner—those intended to preserve democracy and undo classism and elitism—hit the ugly reality of American life. By the 1920s, when the dust began to settle on the effects of the subsequent standardization of medical education that followed the Flexner Report, it was clear that the rational redistribution of well-trained practitioners throughout the country, which Flexner promised, never took place. Instead, the choices of new graduates remained much the same as they had been before: graduates would choose a specialization and then attach themselves to the celebrated city-based hospitals for the larger incomes and regular office hours that they promised.[74] At the same time, according to a 1923 report, many rural practitioners, who had been in practice for over twenty-five years and were primarily graduates of these proprietary schools, had begun to retire or die without a replacement in sight. Without the proprietary schools, medical education became more elitist and the opportunities more unequal than ever before.[75] This was not standardization reform any more than the Ford philosophy in Ford's own hands was Fordism. It was, instead, an early glimpse of a medical capitalism that had all the rigor of efficiency but none of its values.

Flexner realized that the ideology of standardization that he had imposed on medical education had actually only given greater strength to the aristocratic tendencies he had worked so hard against. It had also produced a set of standards so pedagogically rigid and unyielding that they returned students to the rote learning paradigm that Flexner had gone out of his way to excoriate. Nothing about the medical educational system that resulted from his report fit his reformist principles.

Although this disappointing result has largely been (mis)attributed to the monopolistic designs of the AMA, it was similar to what was happening with other standardizing attempts across the country (outside of the exceptional example of the American College of Surgeons). When applied at large scale, efficiency was not a solution to the nascent problems of capitalism—it was its pawn. As Thomas Bonner put it in a biting rebuke to the critiques of Flexner's work in the 1970s and 1980s, the aftereffects of Flexner's report reflected neither Flexner's intentions nor those of the Carnegie Foundation, at least in 1910. But what these late-century critiques did do well, Bonner admitted, was to trace out the inequitable realities of medical education that became the norm in the wake of the Flexner Report.[76] This was probably clearest in terms of the fate of Black medical schools, which Flexner himself exceptionalized in his own work as standing outside of efficiency proper: an extra-political, extra-democratic, extra-efficiency situation that demanded an entirely different kind of solution.

The Black Medical Schools

Flexner was one of the few in the mainstream of the 1910s to devote attention to the Black medical schools. This is not to say, though, that his work is easy reading.[77] On the contrary, Flexner's scarcely two-page discussion of the "Negro medical schools" is packed with the racism of his era. His rationale for training Black physicians rests in not insignificant part on the fact, as he puts it, that "ten million of them live in close contact with sixty million whites" so that "their" diseases were or would become the diseases of their white neighbors if their health was not improved. "Self-protection," he therefore suggests, "not less than humanity offers weighty counsel in this matter." Helping the Black population to modernize their health beliefs and services, then, was "not only for [their] sake, but for ours."[78]

Despite these views, or perhaps because of them, Flexner emerged as a great champion of the schools that he selected for saving: Meharry Medical College in Nashville and Howard University's medical school in Baltimore. He supported them even as his career moved from the Carnegie Foundation to the Rockefeller Foundation, both by defending their continued existence and through the impressive influx of cash and resources that he was able to direct to them.[79]

What is clear, however, is that the general logic that guided Flexner throughout the bulk of the report did not apply to the Black medical schools. The problem for the Black medical schools was not overproduction but rather massive *underproduction*. But even thinking in terms of production provided an impoverished gloss for a much more complex problem. It was certainly true that there were few Black physicians, especially in the South. But also the demand for Black practitioners was purportedly not high: a result both of the sheer absence of and thus unfamiliarity with Black medical practitioners over the preceding decades, as well as the apparent preference for traditional ethnomedical therapies among former slaves and their children and grandchildren, who were supposed to be the Black medical practitioner's keenest clients.[80]

Even though the market transition toward the acceptance of Black medical practitioners would take some time, Flexner considered the matter of increasing the number of Black medical practitioners to be urgent. This was by no means in the same egalitarian spirit that he applied to his other work; he certainly wasn't motivated by anything like W. E. B. Du Bois's vision of a "talented tenth" of Black students who would move into professional and social leadership positions—as medical practitioners in this case—and help guide integrative policies in the future. For Flexner, it was about creating a bulwark of Black physicians who would reduce disease circulating in Black populations with the explicit goal of protecting the white populations with whom they might rub elbows.

In this sense, the characterization of the Black medical schools as underproducing served to situate the Black medical schools as firmly *outside* the norms of standardization—and thus capitalism—that came to underpin the claims of overproduction on which the Flexner Report hung its hat. The problem of the Black medical school was for him an entirely separate issue, made parenthetical from the white mainstream in the ongoing story of American political and economic change. Here, as in the case of the hospital standardization movement, standardization served as yet another form of segregation, if not more outright exclusion.

Indeed, the structure of the Flexner Report renders this tangible. Forming almost a postscript to his nearly two hundred pages of narrative description of the medical school problem, Flexner's brief account of the Black medical schools is wedged into the text as a final chapter, just after a similarly scant treatment of women's medical schools (which served no purpose, he vigorously massaged the truth, because most medical institutions were already coed) and just before the text moves away from narrative altogether and on to a listing of the compiled results of his inspection, in alphabetical order by state.

Of course, to some degree, Flexner's treatment of the Black medical schools as a problem apart from those afflicting the white medical schools reflected the realities of the recent past. The Civil War had ended just fifty years prior, and the legal and social framework of Jim Crow was still strong. Throughout the country, but most explicitly in the South, racism remained the governing norm. The thorny problem of how to integrate the millions whom the Civil War freed from slavery into preexisting political and economic structures had ready articulation in the debates around Black education, most famously articulated in the contrasting views of Booker T. Washington, who favored vocational training and a more gradual course of assimilation, and Du Bois, who posited that educating the most elite and capable of Black students would provide the "thoughtful [people] and trained leadership" needed for the quickest and most effective path toward integration.[81]

While Washington and Du Bois considered how best educational reform might accomplish integration, however, a different tradition associated with Black educational reform played a more critical role in Flexner's characterization of both the problem of Black medical education and its solutions. Though not all of the contemporary Black medical colleges that opened and closed over this period had been founded by white religious or abolitionist groups, the two Flexner chose to support were.[82] Howard University, named for Major General Oliver Otis Howard, a Civil War hero sometimes known as the "Christian General," had been opened on the heels of the war in 1867 by the Congregationalist missionaries the general had kept company with. Meharry was founded "in 1876 by Samuel Meharry and his four brothers in response to an Act of Kindness he had received on a Kentucky road one rainy night—a chance meeting now known as the Salt Wagon Story."[83] This uncomfortably romanticized story of white beneficence certainly suits the preferred flavor of the period, where white philanthropic agents advocated for Black causes. Additional funding from the Methodists gave Meharry, like Howard, a strongly religious flavor. Both medical colleges were run by a predominantly white administration and faculty for several generations after their founding.

It was with these administrations that Flexner met and corresponded during his surveys. In Meharry's case, Flexner spoke of the excellent reputation of its then president Dr. George Hubbard, whose "half century" of devotion "singly to the elevation of the Negro" and proven abilities to "carefully husband" the "slender resources at his command" were cited as reasons for continued investment there.[84] And though Flexner's confidence in Howard University was in part a result of the preexisting support of the Freedmen's Bureau, which had funded its associated hospital, he and Howard's then president, Wilbur Thirkield, seemed to be on a similar wavelength. After reading Flexner's positive summary of Howard, Thirkield wrote to Pritchett:

> I need not say that we are painfully conscious of the limitations of the School . . . in view of the tremendous responsibility that is upon us in the training of the hundreds of Negro physicians in attendance, who are to so largely shape the physical life of the multitudes of [B]lack people of the South. And their physical and moral welfare, as you know, strongly affect the status of the millions of the white race with whom they are, and must inevitably remain, closely related.[85]

Whether to keep Howard in the good graces of the Carnegie Foundation or by dint of his own beliefs, Thirkield was happy to comport to Flexner's views of the purpose of Black medical education. And though, as Todd Savitt's wonderfully detailed look at the Black medical schools explains, philanthropic giving was not immediately forthcoming, by the 1920s, both Meharry and Howard had been the recipients of substantial funds, courtesy of the Rockefeller Foundation, by way of Flexner.[86]

To this line of charitable giving as a solution to Black integration, Du Bois had already given substantial thought. In his seminal 1898 sociological study of race relations in Philadelphia, Du Bois had called out the impulse to charity as evidence of the "same contradictions so often apparent in social phenomena: prejudice and apparent dislike conjoined with widespread and deep sympathy. The same Philadelphian," he continued, "who would not let a Negro work in his store or mill will contribute handsomely to relieve Negroes in poverty and distress."[87] Condemning charity as worse than irrelevant to the larger structural problems of integration, Du Bois called attention to the fact that charitable giving cloaked the desire to resist integration, possibly even to its proponents, in the attire of irreproachable beneficence. In more practical terms, the persistence of this toxic combination of charitable giving in place of integrationist policies created charity itself as an economic necessity. In this way, Black workers in Philadelphia, said Du Bois, were denied access to the social, economic, and political power needed to create, model, and develop an integrated society.

Positioning the problem of Black medical education as uniquely solvable through philanthropic largess rather than structural change reiterated the problems that Du Bois observed. It simulated a social structure in which charity played the leading role while producing an incredibly impoverished model of race relations, and it allowed for, at best, only semiautonomy for Flexner's chosen two Black medical schools, which felt the need to comport themselves according to the expectations of the Carnegie and Rockefeller foundations. It also kept Black medical professionals firmly outside the mainstream of American medicine, although the overt racism of the local medical societies, to whom the AMA had been entrusted all admittance decisions, had already made this exclusion clear by rejecting nearly all Black physicians who applied for membership. And though none of the medical schools could ultimately be said to have affirmed Flexner's goals of "democratic" education as begetting social plasticity, the Flexnerian policy toward the Black medical schools was overtly of the more "aristocratic" sort that Flexner otherwise derided as strengthening, rather than removing, the constraints that kept individuals in their place.

Of course, the Black medical schools have their own individual stories to tell. Savitt reminds us, after all, that neither Meharry nor Howard—nor any of the other medical schools that existed in the period for that matter—produced medical practitioners who were *just* the simple sanitarians that Flexner described, tasked with the protection of the white population from the Black multitudes with whom they would "inevitably remain," as Thirkield had put it, in close contact.[88]

Flexner himself seemed to realize this, relating to Pritchett in 1921 what he had learned from a group of Howard University medical students who had applied for a fellowship to do additional training in the Northeast. As Flexner described it, the explicit purpose of the fellowship, which had been funded by Julius Rosenwald, was to offer additional training to these students so that they "would thus become better teachers in Negro medical schools and more efficient leaders of their own race in public health matters." But the fellowship had a geographical subtext, invisible to readers now but clear at least to Flexner. It was understood, he clarified, that these students would then head south, "to practice medicine and public health among their own people." The problem, Flexner reported to Pritchett, was that not one of the students "intend[ed] to or could be induced" to do this. Instead, they envisioned careers either in the East, where they were already, or in the Northwest.[89]

Black medical students were not, of course, any more conformist to Flexner's systemic requirements regarding distribution than white students were. But his solution was not to recalibrate his approach. As Flexner told Pritchett, the answer was instead to double down on Meharry as the only hope to produce the much-needed Black physicians that could solve the "race problem" in the United States, which was really, as Flexner seemed to see it, a Southern problem.[90]

Flexner's approach to the Black medical schools located them on the outside efficiency's logic, in this way also setting them outside the attendant questions about democracy, egalitarianism, and enfranchisement that he thought standardization—in educational contexts—would answer. In this sense, his attempts to modernize the Black medical schools reinforced their exclusion from that modernity. Unlike the "poor boy," whose fate the implementation of medical educational standards was meant explicitly to improve, the Black medical student was sidelined from the beginning as both untouched and untouchable by the kinds of structural improvements and ideological concerns that drove efficiency reforms more broadly. Here, it was the charity model decried by Du Bois that proliferated, assuring aid to maintain particular Black medical schools as long as they comported themselves appropriately.

5

The Market

The public through universal education is being taught to think, to reason, yet the medical profession today, like the cults, is asking the public to accept goods on faith without investigation; and we claim as a standard science based on reason, not wholly on faith.—G. SHEARMAN PETERKIN, MD, "Ethical Economics," 1919

February 1, 1926, was a rainy Monday in Tucson, Arizona, but the skies were clearing as its citizens made their way through the streets to their evening entertainment. The comedy *We Moderns* was playing at the Rialto. *Bright Lights* was on at the Opera House. The King Vidor drama *His Hour* was being screened at The Lyric Theater, and for the fraternal few, the Knights of Pythias were holding a meeting at the Independent Order of Odd Fellows Hall.[1] None of these, however, were the main draw. This evening, discerning citizens were flocking to the city's high school auditorium to see a traveling spectacle that would have just two performances before moving on to the next town. The hot ticket in town that evening was a community health meeting.

As they toured across the nation according to an itinerary set by planners at the American College of Surgeons, the community health meetings followed a proven formula. The program had much in common with the popular itinerant "medicine shows" of the nineteenth century, where the likes of Harry Houdini and early stars of the bluegrass and country music scene got their start performing between live advertisements for proprietary medical compounds and other wares.[2] It also echoed the antituberculosis crusades launched just as the community health meetings were getting their start—these also featured an easily digestible combination of entertainment, catchy advertisements, and jingles about proper public health care.[3] And it included a righteous dose of the fire and brimstone found in the popular religious revivals of the era, with roaring speeches from a set of "dynamic doctors" damning the debauched "roaring twenties" and prophesying about impending health doom. "Hip pocket flasks, all night dances, necking parties and parked automobiles!" testified one Dr. Allan Craig, enumerating the existential threats to Tucson's younger generation.[4] "Disaster doesn't run into . . . us. We run into disaster!"[5]

Between and around the doctors' sermons, there were motion pictures and musical interludes (this evening's meeting featured local vocalists Mr. and Mrs. William Wheatley and the University of Arizona orchestra), as well as endorsements from local political figures. In Tucson, the ushers were local nurses dressed in the crisp white uniforms of their individual hospitals. In other cities, the matrons sometimes contributed to the musical program. At one meeting in the new Chicago Stadium, a choir of a thousand singing nurses entertained a crowd that packed the venue to the rafters (with standing room, the stadium could accommodate nearly nineteen thousand). With the promise of entertainment like this, the public certainly seemed eager to take part in what one newspaper called the "great game of public health."[6]

In their pageantry and certainly in the addition of motion pictures, these meetings owed much to the public health crusades from which they undoubtedly drew inspiration. But there was one striking difference between those and the community health meetings of the American College of Surgeons. At their events, public health crusaders delivered carefully orchestrated messages about the dire health risks of spitting, not wearing shoes, sharing water cups, or not using mosquito netting—all done up in the advertising vernacular of the day. In Tucson, however, speakers did not bother to translate the risks that germ theory had revealed into real-time, everyday behavioral prescription. Nor did they simply call the public's attention to the health dangers of the world around them—the hookworms lingering in the grass, the mosquitoes waiting to attack.[7] In some ways, as those involved happily admitted, these community health meetings were not about education at all.

Indeed, when these traveling spectacles had begun as a twinkle in the eye of the most prominent hospital standardizers at the American College of Surgeons around 1917, they were intended to "creat[e] and maintain a proper public opinion," or as Charles B. Moulinier, the president of the Catholic Hospital Association and staunch proselytizer of the College's hospital standardizing agenda, put it, their explicit purpose was to "standardize the public mind."[8] Recognizing that the success of the hospital standardization program rested on public buy-in, the College wanted to inculcate meeting-goers not with helpful tips for maintaining public health but with the desire to trust their health to a standardized practitioner practicing modern, standardized medicine in a modern, standardized hospital. This meant selling the idea that uniformity and consistency were *medical* values that consumers ought to hold for the same reasons these qualities were valued in other aspects of life.

Unusual though it was in the context of the medical crusades of the period to sell something so esoteric as a "standard," it was not strange to think that standards themselves might have real consumer appeal. After all, Henry Ford had demonstrated the egalitarian value of standardization for consumers with his Model T, which was just reaching the height of its popularity when the health meetings were taking off. It was well understood that the standardization of parts had driven down the cost of manufacturing to such an extent that automobile ownership moved swiftly from luxury good to something well within the reach of the middle-class buyer.[9] In other parts of daily life, mass production had made standardized objects affordable and increasingly common—objects like washing machines, refrigerators, stoves, dishwashers, and radios were slowly establishing themselves as the backdrop to the domestic every day.[10]

And sell the standard they did. From a basic public relations approach that began with placing editorials in newspapers and magazines across the country, the College grew more ambitious and sophisticated. It opened its membership meetings to the public, padding pedagogical content with an increasing number of entertaining interludes. Before long, it was conducting a full schedule of community meetings with large crowds and an even larger audience that listened in on the radio.

Just as the College's methods evolved over time, so too did its message. For although audiences were still receptive to standardization as a medical value in and of itself in the late 1910s, interest seemed to dwindle by the early 1920s. And thus the themes subtly shifted to emphasizing not the standards themselves but the salubrious impact these standards would have on one's own personal well-being. From there, it was just a hop, skip, and a jump to a familiar paean for modern medicine as an intrinsically curative, lifesaving venture. This was the portrait of medicine painted by the American College of Surgeons by the late 1920s and early 1930s.

The marketing of standardized medicine described in this chapter indicates one kind of inevitable outcome of the hospital standardization program of the College, which needed a market in order to survive and thrive. It also manifests how the College shifted its language around health to sell this commodity, following in this way the ethos of an era as it moved from a fascination with standardization to a fascination with personalized, particularized, unique health care services. Almost unwittingly, then, the College assisted in the arrival of a discourse of modern medicine that would be used against standardization. Over at the American Medical Association (AMA), the modern medicine that standardization built was being reinvented during the 1930s. Rather than sell the public on the value of standardization as a force for innovation, self-expression, or modernity, the AMA would now disparage it as something that overrode autonomy, disregarded individuality, and stultified personal difference, all in the name of what had become a dirty word: efficiency.

Spreading the Word

At a conference in 1917, just as the hospital standardization program of the American College of Surgeons was beginning in earnest, the conversation turned to the question of how to attract the public to its newly standardized hospitals. One of Moulinier's favored marketing methods was to follow the common practice of both soliciting and crafting strong testimonials to be printed in newspapers and magazines across the nation. It was a simple plan, requiring only that the College "get some of the most keen, attractive writers in this country who write for the various magazines, to prepare articles on this subject for the *Saturday Evening Post, Collier's* and a few others of the world-noted magazines."[11] Moulinier sent a note to John Bowman, the director of the American College of Surgeons, suggesting that the College adopt this approach, and Bowman agreed. Over the next two years, a steady stream of glowing articles appeared in the nonmedical press, explaining the hospital standardization program and its benefit for the public.

One of the first of these came from Bowman himself in an article in the June 2, 1918, Sunday edition of the *New York Times*. The front page of the broadsheet was all about the war: the German army had gained six miles, turning west toward Paris in an apparent attempt to surprise the Allies. This left the American troops, declared General Bridges, the head of the Special British Military Mission to the United States, to "hold the balance between defeat and victory."[12]

Bowman's article, seventy-two pages later in the weekly magazine section, also talked about the conflict, but he saw in its violence an opportunity for a victory lap. A "standardization plan launched by the American College of Surgeons before the war," he wrote, was "now developing for [the] benefit of soldiers" on the front line in France.[13] He continued,

> Where did the army get its medical efficiency of this character? Back of it all is a big idea, a "vision," a determination on the part of the leading surgeons of this continent which found expression four years ago. There was no world war then. But these surgeons met in Washington and with the highest seriousness that ever comes to men they asked: "Is the best surgery too good for the humblest patient? ... Is there the slightest reason why we should not take hold with all the strength in us and force the right sort of ideals in surgery to come true all over our continent?" That meeting in Washington was the beginning of the American College of Surgeons. It was the beginning of a great idea which today saves the life of many a soldier as well as the lives of untold thousands of laymen.[14]

If the beloved doughboys made it home in one piece, Bowman seemed to be saying, it was because the far-seeing College had started a medical standardization effort back while Archduke Franz Ferdinand was still enjoying his carriage rides. In a war infamous for the deadliness of trench warfare, mustard gas, aerial attacks, and machine guns, standardization was achieving its own medico-martial victory.

In careful detail, Bowman explained for the reader how this transformation had come about. First, there was the keeping of thorough medical records, thereby allowing doctors to know the "exact facts" of a patient's case and track patient outcomes. Then, to best "profit" from these exact facts, hospitals were organizing regularly scheduled staff meetings at which doctors and surgeons would discuss their cases. Here, diagnostic and therapeutic choices could be measured against outcomes, and those with the worst outcomes could be called to task and forced to reform or, failing that, resign. Finally, there was the laboratory, a critical, modern hospital feature to which all doctors, now under the close scrutiny of their peers, would be "sharply incentivized" to turn so as to avoid the embarrassment that came with diagnoses that were "mere guesswork" and the expulsion that would inevitably come should that guesswork lead them consistently astray.[15]

Long after the war had ended, Bowman and other members of the College continued to write editorials in the same vein, each tying the College's standardizing work to contemporary events or offering slants acutely aligned to the leanings of a particular publication's readership. A 1920 article in *World's Work*, a business-centric magazine that defiantly bucked journalism's muckraking trend, assured its readers that the American College of Surgeons was not interested in "up-lift" or "welfare work," nor was its standardization program "a sentimental betterment affair of any description."[16] Instead, its minimum standard was a guarantee of accountability and an "insistence upon competence on the part of the doctor" through practices such as keeping case records, holding staff meetings, and establishing laboratory facilities.[17] Furthermore, the writer emphasized, these changes had come from within the profession itself, safeguarding it against the imposition of government regulation.

Testimonials from successful personages followed. An unnamed surgical source described how the College had "revolutionized the practice of medicine in Baltimore," and Henry Pritchett, whose Carnegie Foundation had been quietly backing the College's efforts (to the tune of $105,000) for several years, gushed that "an advance normally to be expected in twenty years ha[d] come in three."[18] In many ways, it was an apt companion piece to another testimonial from a decade earlier that appeared in *World's Work*, in which Edgar Allan Forbes heaped praise on Abraham Flexner, applauding his hard-nosed approach to the streamlining of medical schools.[19]

Even as it continued to place articles in newspapers and magazines, however, the American College of Surgeons started to diversify its marketing strategy. In April 1919, the College opened the afternoon and evening sessions of its hospital standardization conference in Portland, Oregon, to the general public, with an invitation printed in the local papers. The meeting was held at a local high school, but if the setting was indicative of the College's attempt to find common health ground between clinical and lay populations, the talks were not. The afternoon session primarily featured lackluster speeches on the College's signature activity: the hospital standardization program. Following an introduction by Bowman, several surgeons took turns explaining the importance of standardization, offering specific details about the College's tripartite intervention: case records, monthly staff meetings, and clinical laboratories.

The evening meeting began at 8 p.m., with Moulinier reading an endorsement of the College's "high aims" and extending invitation to the citizens of Portland to join in the waves of "enthusiasm" that he claimed were already "displayed throughout the country over the proposed standardization plans."[20] This was the rhetorical highlight of the evening. Compared to the subsequent

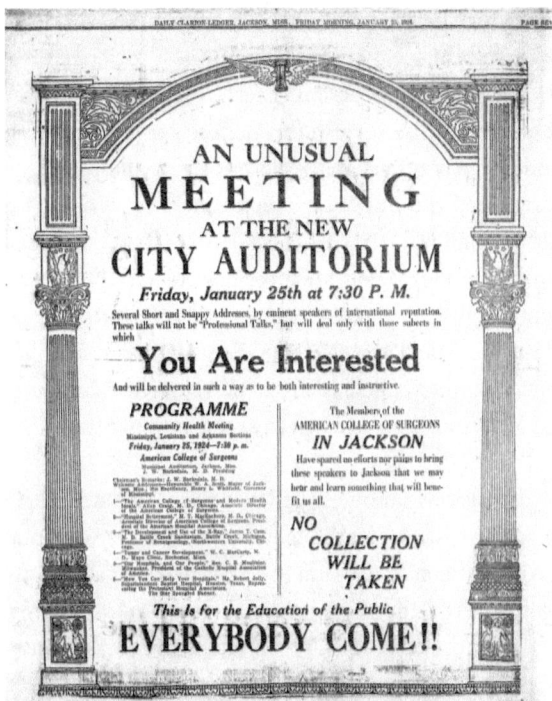

FIGURE 5.1. A newspaper announcement for the American College of Surgeons Community Health Meeting in Jackson, Mississippi. *Daily Clarion-Ledger*, January 25, 1924.

efforts to engage the public, the event was quite dry, with not a whiff of entertainment to be had.

Gradually, the meetings began to improve their staid formats, starting with a bit of pageantry borrowed from the College's annual congresses. The College's bronze mace put in appearances, typically in the hands of the "military mace bearer" who placed it before the gathering during multiple "eulogies" of the College and its work.[21] The "velvet-faced," scarlet-tasseled fellowship costume, the same that College critic Philip Mills Jones had in earlier years mocked as ridiculously pretentious, was also taken out of its mothballs and draped across the shoulders of the College dignitaries.[22] And the invitations got showier, incorporating different fonts and typefaces for visual appeal as well as decorative borders and promises to deliver talks only on health matters in which "You Are Interested," as one advertisement in a Jackson, Mississippi, paper announced in 1924 (figure 5.1).[23]

At the same time, the meetings acquired a more local flavor. In these early years, the meetings were concentrated on the southern edge of Canada and in American states west and south of the American College of Surgeons headquarters in Chicago, since these were the communities where the College felt its hold was weakest. Employing the tenets of what we might now call lean management, the College tasked the local medical and surgical societies with putting together and participating in the program of each meeting, in this way increasing the local sense of enfranchisement in the College's activities. After all, standardization was not strictly a national issue but rather hundreds of very local problems that required the buy-in of practitioners for whom the College's program still held little allure.

Thus, outreach took on two prongs. The state meetings created the opportunity for the College to enfranchise local physicians and surgeons working at local hospitals, so they would embrace its goals. And the community health meetings allowed it to convince ordinary people to patronize the standard hospital, the critical work that Moulinier had referred to as the "standardizing" of the public's minds.[24]

The American College of Surgeons genuinely believed that standard hospitals were better hospitals, so efforts to bring this news to the public were not disingenuous. But it needed the standard hospital to sell; it needed patients to choose this option. And this was the aim of its publicizing and enfranchising work: to serve the practical purpose of drumming up and guaranteeing business for these hospitals.

It was not an easy sell. Though wide agreement existed around the sentiment that standard care was tantamount to best care, standardization was an expensive and time-consuming process for hospitals, despite the fact that the required standards remained minimal and unchanging over the early years of the program. Indeed, this was one of the barriers to entry that could make standardization so disenfranchising. Building laboratories cost money, and maintaining and storing records necessitated more work for physicians, more space for storage, and more staff. Hospitals in the less College-influenced areas of the country needed more incentive to take part in the hospital standardization program. Specifically, they needed to know that they would make back the money they spent on standardizing through an uptick in patients, preferably of the paying variety, who would choose their hospitals *because* they were standard. In real ways, this characterized the hospital standardization movement more broadly as one that was for and about an already enfranchised population of people who could and would appreciate the value of a standard and be willing to pay for it.

A major coup for the College came in 1921, when the American Railway Association agreed to have its membership use College-approved hospitals exclusively, for all but the most emergent cases. The physician and spokesperson for the American Railway Association, Daniel Dunott, was invited to the College's hospital conference that year to spell out the weightiness of this partnership. Since the railroads of member companies covered "two hundred and eighty-four thousand miles of railroad in the United States and Canada," and since accidents could happen at any point along these hundreds of thousands of miles, he explained, the American Railway Association physicians regularly used about "four-fifths of the hospitals of the country." The railroad association's commitment to College-approved hospitals surely provided added incentive for hospitals nationwide to standardize: the College had struck a lucrative deal with a large, widely distributed, and uniquely accident-prone workforce.[25]

But just as meaningful, if not more so, the College suggested, was the pressure that local citizens and communities could put on their own local hospitals to standardize. To this end, community health meetings featured speeches about how "the people of" Tucson, Pittsburgh, Little Rock, Des Moines, or wherever they were that day "would be helped by the work of the College" and how these same citizens could, in turn, give back. Collaboration, then, at the local level was starting to become the name of the game.

Indeed, almost from the beginning, the American College of Surgeons took care to customize its message toward local communities and their decision-makers. Speakers at the community health meeting in Ottawa, Canada, in 1923 congratulated the city on "having such a fine auditorium in connection with its high school and such a splendid orchestra."[26] In Tucson in 1926, the College's founder, Franklin Martin, admired the wonders of the Arizona desert lifestyle, claiming its health effects to be so great that it was the place where the "wornout batteries of the east come to be recharged." Its health-giving climate was matched, he added, by surgeons so excellent that "you will not hold [your surgeons] here always, for many cities of the east, where these batteries are being worn out, are looking to these surgeons." What could Tucson do to make sure that it would keep its surgeons local? It must provide standardized hospitals for these excellent standardized surgeons to work in, of course, which meant banding together and making the commitment *as a community* to patronize only these hospitals.[27]

Over the years of the community health meetings, but especially in their earliest incarnations, spectacular surgeons were found everywhere the College went, singled out alongside other points of local pride—the special features of the land, the buildings, the music, the entertainment, the people of each and every city. Truly *nobody* did it better, according to the patter of the community health speakers, than the citizens of [fill in the blank]. Though the increasing crowds and enthusiasm for the health meetings indicated the success of this strategy, it did occasionally backfire, as in Brooklyn in 1928, when, much to the chagrin of the reporter from the *Brooklyn Daily Eagle* who covered the event, the obviously "out-of-town speakers" kept referring to the Brooklyn borough president as the mayor of New York City, who was not in attendance.[28]

Such moments of questioning press coverage were rare, however. In fact, the few skeptics that did put their criticism into print generally hailed from within the medical profession itself, often to voice disgust with what they viewed as the College's propagandizing efforts. Claiming in 1933 that the College had hired "experienced newspapers writers" to prepare articles that were then "multigraphed and distributed to the press of the whole country," the medical columnist James Brady accused the group of having engineered "front page publicity and flattering personal mention" with the specific intent to raise its own—not medicine's—public image.[29]

Brady was of course correct. It was common, especially as time went on, for the same laudatory texts on the College and its work to appear simultaneously in different local newspapers, appended as appropriate to the details of local connections: local venues used by "prominent" nationally known visiting surgeons, local surgeons elevated to the ranks of fellowship, or local hospitals added to the College's increasingly coveted approved list.[30]

Likewise, it was an open secret that the College worked hard to get local newspapers, especially early on, to note and properly render its goals and activities. The local newspapers in Spokane, Washington, for example, had given the College a hard time about running content concerning the community health meetings there in the late 1920s. So it was rather triumphantly that Malcolm MacEachern—who represented the American College of Surgeons and whose work in hospital management was so influential that he later earned the honorific "Mr. Hospital"—reported that these same papers had invited the College back, asking that the health meetings that they had initially refused to cover a few years before now be offered to all the city's high schools.[31]

The press and the College had created their own mutual appreciation society. After a 1926 community health meeting in Montreal, the omnipresent MacEachern publicly congratulated the city's newspapers for their excellent reporting on the College's work, noting that the College did not need "to aid the papers to get accurate reports," as was the case in nearly every other city the College visited. Then, in a demonstration of the kind of ace reporting MacEachern was talking about, the *Montreal Gazette* carried this praise at the tail end of the College's visit there, proudly informing its readership of the accuracy with which it conveyed the College messaging.[32]

If the increase in crowds and enthusiasm for the community health meetings could be considered a barometer of the success of these behind-the-scenes marketing machinations, they were clearly working. In 1922, Franklin Martin noted that the community health meetings reliably had audiences of between 500 and 3,000. In that "last meeting we had in that little town in Ontario, of less than 100,000 population, we had an attendance of 2200," he crowed, which meant that "the speakers, including the mayor of the town, had to fight to get into the hall because the crowd was so deep they could not get in otherwise."[33] Especially for the purposes of reporting ahead to cities still to come on the road trip, these kinds of optics were phenomenal. Popularity begot popularity.

A decade later, crowds had grown far larger. MacEachern, speaking on the eve of a community health meeting in St. Louis, Missouri, told colleagues at the board of regents meeting there that they expected "5,000 or more" at the meeting.[34] Two years after that, in Oklahoma City,

> they began coming to the Warner Theatre at six o'clock for the program which was to begin at seven-thirty, and we had to send several thousand home. In Salt Lake City we took the Mormon Tabernacle and put in 10,000 altogether, and then we had to open the assembly hall for an overflow; and yet a couple of thousand were sent home. In Spokane we were prepared for an overflow, but even then we had to turn several thousand away. According to a lady from Spokane, whom I met on the street later, 15,000 were turned away who couldn't get in.[35]

By the 1930s, the College was not just offering community health meetings but also preparing speeches for schools (in 1934, it covered "37 senior high schools" while "on the road") and giving presentations to Rotarians, Elks, Moose, Odd Fellows, Knights (often of Pythias, perhaps of the Maccabees, certainly of Columbus), Sons and Daughters of the American Revolution and of the Civil War, some Shriners or Owls, and a scattering of Masons.[36]

To expand its reach even further, the American College of Surgeons also began to broadcast its meetings over the radio waves. In Los Angeles in 1934, seven thousand attended a massive meeting, while an estimated half a million tuned in over the wireless.[37] In October 1933, as part of the larger schedule of activities for Chicago's Century of Progress exposition (just weeks before the *Graf Zeppelin* arrived to stun exposition visitors by hovering around the southern end of Lake Michigan), the College held its international congress, adding speeches made there, for the benefit of the average citizen, to NBC's radio offerings. Every day from October 9–13, between 3:15 p.m. and 3:30 p.m., the residents of western Massachusetts could listen to prominent surgeons talk about "the control and cure of cancer," "the crippled child," and "your personal responsibility for health."³⁸ Though the schedules varied, the same was true in Connecticut and the countless other communities in the northeast that also added the broadcasts to their local radio offerings.³⁹

The Message

The College's success was largely due to its effective marketing campaigns, but it needed substance to match. It could only get so far on a diet of self-aggrandizing claims of oversold assembly halls and high school auditoriums and laudatory newspaper articles celebrating the College as "conceived in idealism, nurtured in altruism and matured in utilitarianism."⁴⁰ It needed to do more than convince the public that it was a high-minded organization or, as time wore on, that standards were a worthy pursuit no matter the subject matter. Indeed, given the well-known insularity and disunity of medicine over the first decades of the twentieth century, these sorts of claims might even have come across as ironic, or at least transparently self-serving.⁴¹ But it mattered relatively little, in any case, what the people who came to hear its experts believed was true about medicine more generally. The American College of Surgeons wanted audiences to leave the meetings with the kind of commitment to "standard" medicine that would actually see them choosing standard hospitals and standard surgeons for their care. In short, the College needed its audiences to resituate themselves vis-à-vis this new system of health care.

Initially, the community health meeting fare was less successful in achieving this goal. In 1920, the College had a small program and visited just a handful of cities, arranging for three or four talks from a team that was anchored by heavyweights from Chicago headquarters—Martin, Bowman, and often Moulinier—plus a rotating lineup of other speakers. A local politician, religious figure, or celebrity generally opened the meetings, introducing the College and calling up the first visitor to speak. The talks followed a simple format: introduce the tenets of hospital standardization and then invoke the relationship between public health improvement and standardization.

Though they continued to recite the details of the College's hospital standardization program, these talks—like Bowman's editorial in the *New York Times*—explained the College's turn toward the patient as the centerpiece of its program. Over the first year or so of meetings, the talks largely construed the patient in the abstract, describing how a patient ought to be and act in relation to health care, just as Bowman's editorials had. In one typical talk in Phoenix in 1920, both Franklin Martin and Frederic Besley, a College member and chief medical consultant of the American Expeditionary Forces, recycled and co-opted the patriotic patter of the recently ended war to suggest that it was the duty of every good citizen to see the doctor. "You are all interested in having A1 citizens in Arizona," Besley said, intoning the highest level of military fitness to an audience in Phoenix. "But you cannot have A1 citizens unless you have healthy citizens. And you cannot have healthy citizens unless you are cooperating and working with your physicians and surgeons."[42]

The patient that Martin and Besley conjured up was one that would, as Bowman attempted to drive home in his speech, accept the expertise of the medical community, allowing doctors and surgeons to protect their health much as the police offered protection for "the right to walk the streets freely" or the law protected the right "to own property," as College officials put it. And what the College desired, as the *Salt Lake City Tribune* wrote, was the "cooperation of an awakened public" to accept the authority of medical practitioners to "protect" a person's health and, more particularly, to patronize College-sanctioned hospitals and surgeons. It was, the speakers told their audiences from Phoenix to Boise to Pittsburgh to Butte, nothing less than their patriotic duty.[43]

A year later, in 1921, the College started to make significant alterations to its messaging. The first order of business seemed to be making the talks more entertaining, mapping them increasingly onto both the recently extinct "medicine shows" of the late nineteenth century and the health campaigns growing around them. Not only did they increasingly cover issues of interest to the general public—Prohibition, pregnancy and childbirth, the popular new technology of X-rays, common diseases—but they also became more performative and more vividly illustrated and presented. In "pep star" Allan Craig, the College had its own Will Rogers. Craig used humorous asides and had a penchant for folksy turns of phrase. His talk "Adding Years to Your Life" was a particular hit, especially for its colorful condemnation of the American youth of the 1920s. Youngsters, it seemed, were a real thorn in Craig's side, or at least that is what his condemnation of their late nights, illicit alcohol use, and abhorrent fondness for jazz seemed to suggest. The seemingly abstemious audiences did not seem to mind. Indeed, the popularity of these talks suggested that meeting-goers were not the hedonistic libertines, flappers, or other rebellious malcontents of F. Scott Fitzgerald's *The Great Gatsby*. They were also not the poor working class or the disenfranchised post-Reconstruction Black communities of the South or W. E. B. Du Bois's "talented tenth." The community health meetings were aimed squarely at the solid, stolid "silent majority" of the American middle class, on whose patronage health care increasingly turned.[44]

On the back of his success in painting such a deliciously unflattering portrait of the youth of the roaring twenties, Craig would also be pressed into

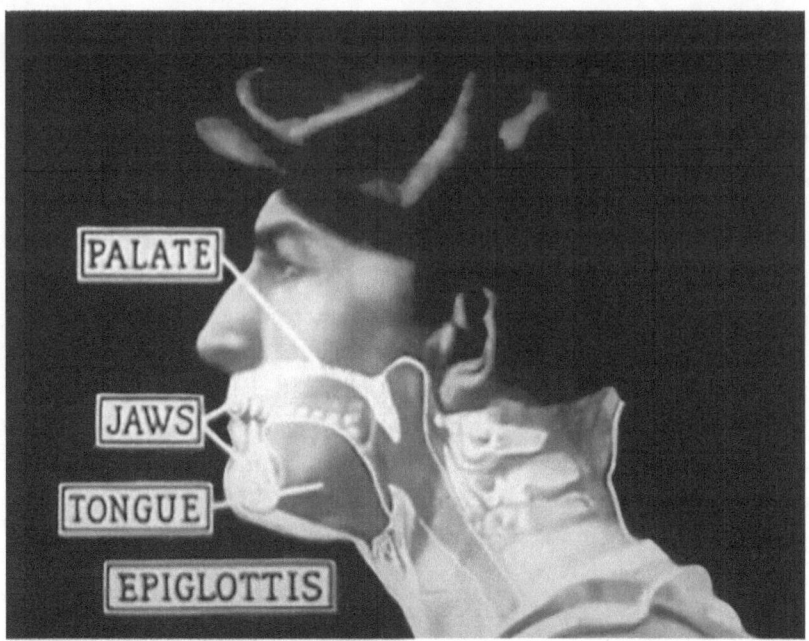

FIGURE 5.2. A still from the 1926 film *How the Fires of the Body Are Fed*, a popular feature at American College of Surgeons meetings during the late 1920s.

service as narrator for one of the College's most popular additions, a 1926 film called *How the Fires of the Body Are Fed*, which detailed the process of digestion (figure 5.2).[45] Craig's obvious rapport with the crowd shone through on at least one occasion when he narrated a double feature, *How the Fires of the Body Are Fed* and *One Scar or Many*, on smallpox vaccination. Afterward, an anti-vaxxer stood up in the audience to call foul on Craig's pro-vaccination talk.

"'Let me ask you a question,' [the heckler] cried. 'Would you dare to give a written statement of safety to every person you vaccinate?' 'You bet I would,'" Craig shot back, apparently never having met a vaccine he didn't like. With the crowd cheering him on, Craig then invited the heckler, a Mr. Reimers, up onto the stage to debate. Amid the "boos and shouts" directed at Reimers as he took the stage, a pleased Craig "stood smilingly" by—happy, as the newspaper later put it, to "accept the judgment of the audience as sufficient vindication" of the rightness of his views.[46] This audience, as far as the College was concerned, had been effectively standardized.

As time went on, the College's productions expanded, filling at least two and sometimes up to three hours, during which, Martin claimed, the audience remained "at the end of the seat" and "eat[ing] up what we have to say to them."[47]

Local politicians, who used to merely introduce the speakers from the American College of Surgeons, now served as warm-up acts before the main event. Local celebrities and "dignitaries" would appear at events in nonspeaking roles, arranging themselves over the platform to survey the crowds and listen to the message.[48] Local musicians entertained the crowds, while a rotating slate of movies provided entertaining *and* purportedly educational interludes. Further accoutrements included the singing of national anthems (of the United States or Canada, depending on the venue) as well as "local nurses" who frequently showed up en masse to the events in some variant of the "natty white uniforms" that graced the 1922 Asheville, North Carolina, meeting. These uniformed nurses were especially welcome at the events, thought one reporter, for the addition of an atmosphere that "harmonized well" with the health messages the College was delivering.[49]

While these additions no doubt had a hand in increasing attendance and drumming up enthusiasm for the meetings, the problem to be solved was not getting people to go to the meetings, which they were increasingly inclined to do, but to the standardized hospitals. A shifted tactic in nascent form came already in the 1920 version of Bowman's talk on hospital standardization. Taking a folksier approach than in his editorials, Bowman began by emphasizing the more tangible and personal aspects of cooperation with its health endeavors. This was not just the abstracted patient's health or the return to health of "our boys over there," it was *your own* personal health that hung in the balance.

"Some day it may happen that . . . you have a pain in your stomach," he began, "and you have to go [to the hospital]. On that day you are going to take a serious inventory and among the questions that you are going to ask yourself is this: Have I a right to be well?"[50]

It is unclear whether this was really the question foremost in the minds of audience members as they imagined their own (stomach) pain-addled selves contemplating hospitalization. However, the intonation of one's own personal well-being and the newly specific, newly visceral ties of personal health to the College's standardization activities set the tone for future community health meetings as they developed over the next several years.

What followed in Bowman's talk in 1920 remained true to the talks of that year: a detailed accounting of the College's hospital standardization program, featuring the ever-present need to "cooperate" with the program's vision by patronizing only standard hospitals. But the reference to personal health quickly caught on as the hook to convince people that choosing a standard hospital was not just about duty or the health of the public in general. At stake was the alleviation of one's own "pain," in the stomach or elsewhere. Standards suddenly had specific and personal implications.

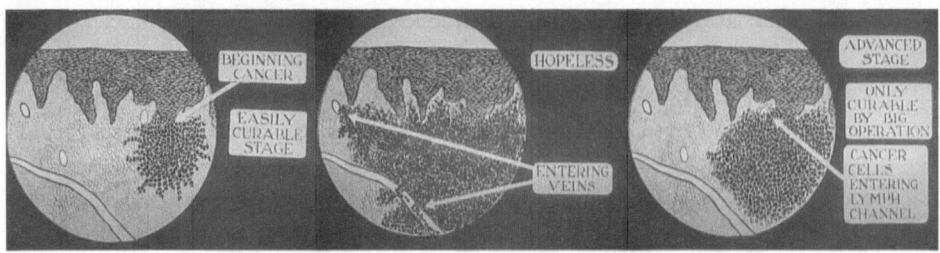

FIGURE 5.3. The stages of cancer as depicted in the 1921 Cancer Society film *The Reward of Courage*, which was shown as part of the American College of Surgeons community health meetings throughout the 1920s.

One of the most important ways in which the College developed this theme came through the addition of talks on cancer. From the start, cancer's high public profile (or, rather, the widespread dread of the disease) made it a reliable health meeting draw. Cancer also perfectly illustrated the new messaging: not only was public cooperation with hospital standardization a civic or patriotic duty, but patronizing doctors early and often was itself of critical and curative personal importance in one's own fight against this most feared disease.

The parade of cancer experts began to cross the health meeting stages in early 1921, each reliably dropping the bombshell that cancer was completely curable (figure 5.3). This was not because treatments had improved. Indeed, as Besley first indicated in 1920 and others repeated well into the 1930s, the treatment of cancer remained limited to the burn, cut, and poison regimen available at the time—namely, radium, X-rays, surgery, and an array of caustics.[51]

And in fact, these speakers typically doubled back on their curative claims, admitting in one manner or another that technically there was no medical "cure" for cancer (as another College speaker rather dubiously explained this double-talk in 1932, cancer was a "biologic and not a medical problem" and thus, logically, not one that could "be cured by medicine").[52]

Instead, the cure for cancer that the College speakers had in mind was a more bureaucratic one that standard medicine was especially well equipped to provide: early detection. Curing cancer, they said, was singularly a question of putting one's body in the hands of a doctor not when one had symptoms, for then it was often too late, but *immediately*.

Why not join a "birthday society"? Martin posed this question to an audience that had just listened to his curable cancer talk in Lincoln, Nebraska, in early 1922. Though this was not actually something that existed (yet), Martin filled the crowd in on his vision: a "body of people who would make it a practice to be examined at least once a year in order to determine if anything was wrong." It was the perfect practice, he said, for those interested in "curing" themselves of the cancer they did not yet have. "At least," Moulinier piled on to Martin's message in Lincoln, "give your body the same care that you give your car. Even," he wryly added, "if it's a Ford."[53] Indeed, for those who did not "cooperate" and give their bodies at least the annual overhauls their cars received, the price might be death. One in fourteen people, after all, would get cancer, the College experts noted. And the prevalence was only increasing; there was a chance that *you—you* in the audience right now, the speakers suggested— already have it but just don't realize.[54]

The College augmented this message with another theme that it sprinkled into its talks: the trustworthiness of College-certified medicine and medical practitioners. College speakers claimed that their object—to visit the doctor early and often—ran counter to the economic interests of the physician. They could not have been guided by financial gain, which had been the well-known bedrock of medical reform activities a mere decade earlier, they implied. Their motivation was instead simple altruism. Indeed, in a 1927 speech to a health meeting crowd gathered in Decatur, Illinois, Herman Bundeson, the health commissioner for Chicago, raised and then debunked the claim that "we are merely publicity agents for physicians." Nothing could be further from the truth, he insisted, since periodic physical examinations brought in only a measly $10 a visit, while a "disease or illness permitted to run" its course would bring in far more.[55]

By the time the community health meetings reached Tucson in 1926, altruism had been joined by transparency. A value strongly associated with standardization anyway, transparency here seemed to some explicitly manifested in the choice of films the College showed. After having viewed *How the Fires of the Body Are Fed*, a journalist for the *Arizona Daily Star* opined that "it was the fact that the film "literally . . . rent asunder" the "veil of secrecy that was wont to shroud the science of medicine since the days of Aesculapius" that ultimately made the film newsworthy.[56] This view, perhaps planted in the minds of the journalists by the College itself, echoed through other papers that reviewed the film. For in freely demonstrating not only what the interior of the human body looked like but also how it functioned, the journalist saw the very essence of what the "worldrenowned savants" who brought the community health meetings to town were all about. This was a group that was willing to take "the public into their confidence [to invite] it into a glorious partnership in the battle for better health."[57]

This sense of collaboration also extended to the advice the College's speakers gave about a growing variety of everyday health situations over the years. This was not, as we might see it now, a situation in which every inch of the body increasingly became subject to medicine's logic. It was instead taken as proof of the moral high ground of medicine more generally. Sharing secrets showed not only a readiness to tear down the "veils of secrecy" that kept medical knowledge from the public. It also showed a willingness to give up the profits that would come from the secrecy of medical knowledge, even to the point of running themselves out of business.

So, when physician Loyal Shoudy told health meeting attendees in Berkeley, California, in 1935 that death from sunstroke was often caused by the victim drinking too much water to alleviate the condition—a situation called "water intoxication"—he was effectively giving away the real cure for sunstroke for free. One should, he advised, not drink water but "swallow some salt in some palatable form instead" to treat the condition. In offering this advice, he was performatively forgoing the fee he would normally receive for his clinical expertise and for his purveying of salt to the victims of sunstroke who came into his care.[58] This, the College repeatedly emphasized, was merely standardized medicine's way. Unique among enterprises, College speakers claimed, medicine had for "twenty-three centuries" provided "unselfish service to humanity," giving away the secrets that other businesses had jealously guarded.[59]

These new foci evinced more than just a new tactic in efforts to persuade the public to get on board with its programs. Conflating the American College of Surgeons with the medical profession—what Brady had so detested—established the College as the standard-bearer for medicine more generally. It produced itself as the right organization to distinguish the good practitioner from the bad and the legitimate practices from quackery.

Cynics might say that it achieved this trustworthy state primarily by continually appropriating more and more of medicine until suddenly its purview was the health of the American public itself. And indeed, it was true, the American College of Surgeons enjoyed increasing, unprecedented power over the two decades of its meetings, and the anointment of those practitioners and institutions who were members and partners became an increasingly necessary step for their economic viability and professional legibility. Medicine was only medicine when it was College-certified.

Yet, the College's health meetings also reflected the underlying tension that had guided both its own and other medical standardizing efforts. Too much control would have spelled its rejection as a standardizing body because of the too-thorough and thus anti-efficiency autocracy that this would imply. But too little control over medicine, experience suggested, would result in the lack of size and authority necessary to make and enforce standards. The attempt to find the balance between the extremes of populism and autocracy in the efficiency discussion had resulted in the rather odd but workable "democracy" of the College's standardization program. This manifested itself in the community health meetings in an equally awkward commitment to folksy talk, grassroots politics, community collaboration, transparency, and altruism. All of which required, first and foremost, buy-in to the notion that standard medicine was the only medicine and standard hospitals the only hospitals.

Whether intentional or not, the College's co-opting of diseases like cancer offered a rhetoric of medicine and the personal stakes associated with it that had not previously existed in any cohesive way. Out of a need to get people to patronize standard hospitals, the College ultimately tapped into, and helped to flesh out, a language of health care that connected the infrastructural and institutional successes of the profession—its standardization—directly to the well-being of each and every individual, while also creating and celebrating a medical backstory of altruism and unselfish service to humankind. This was a far cry from the rhetoric of medicine not even a generation earlier. The College had made good use of human vulnerability, implying by a series of associations that failure to support a standard hospital would result in personal ill health and possibly even death. This message was critical to its legacy and helped to shape what we regard as health care and our need for it today. More to the point, it became, in turn, absolutely critical to the discussion of health care in the next decade, although in a way that the College had not intended—namely, as the American Medical Association's rationale to resist attempts to "standardize" the health care marketplace.

Conclusion

The American College of Surgeons continued to press the relationship between personal health and standard medicine over the remainder of the 1920s and into the 1930s, proclaiming transparency and unselfish service to be the values that underlay all its activities. As the twenties roared along, however, the College found itself somewhat floundering, not because it was struggling to meet its goals but because it had met them rather too well. As early as 1930, it seemed to some "no longer necessary to use great persuasion or stress" to get people to enter a hospital or to choose a standard hospital for their treatment, as the physician and College fellow Carl von Neupert put it. There was now, instead, "distinct demand" for the standard hospital.[60]

Outgoing president J. Bentley Squier echoed this message in 1933. Even in a time of economic depression, he said, medical practitioners never had to "fear that the supply of health we are able to produce will ever overtop the demand." In an explicit reversal of the situation earlier in the century, the College had produced a situation in which demand for medicine seemed unquenchable, so much so that while the rest of the country suffered the consequences of the Great Depression, medicine purportedly continued to thrive. It had become a necessity to Americans—though, as some at the time keenly observed, these Americans were still quite a distinct and specific group: the "silent majority" that the College had appealed to.[61] Citing the novel position of medicine as so essential as to be critical whatever the economic situation, Squier went on to say that "the only tangible asset" that people retained in a depression, "was health." Therefore, he concluded, "there will always be a strong market for such wares."[62]

At a bit of a loss as to what to do next, the College sought new marketing strategies during the 1930s. College speakers began to turn increasing attention to another rhetorical tack familiar to us today: the notion of medicine as spectacular, a thing of "wonders" and "miracles." The famous Charles Mayo told crowds in Pittsburgh in 1933 that a "death ray" supposedly being developed by the US military to "sink battleships" and "defeat armies" was actually already in place in medicine in the form of "radium, X-rays and various forms of electric waves" that took as their enemy that implacable menace, bacteria.[63]

Increasingly, the College began to shift away from associating standardization and other bureaucratic measures with specific and personal health and associated instead its community health meetings with displays of surgical prowess. Newspapers gamely described the activities of the community health meetings alongside depictions and descriptions of miraculous surgical cures, whether or not these were directly associated with the College. In 1935, the "deft use of a surgeon's knife" was extending a child's leg, which had been shortened by infantile paralysis, by two and half inches, miraculously making whole what disease had once taken away.[64] Reports of another miraculous surgical work, this time in 1931, accompanied descriptions of a health meeting in Berkeley. Here readers were treated to the story of a little girl just having undergone brain surgery that saved her from "a certain fate of blindness, delinquency, and feeble-mindedness," restoring her to "normal development and," the article reported, "perhaps even genius" (figure 5.4).[65]

At the accompanying community health meeting, Bowman Crowell, associate director of the American College of Surgeons, let the thousands assembled on that day in on the "seven wonders of medicine": some familiar to us now, some less so. These were, he said, "immunity, anesthesia and analgesia, antisepsis and asepsis, knowledge of food values, light and ventilation, organotherapy and, of course, periodic health examinations."[66] Modern medicine, he told the public, had arrived. And it was not just preventive or curative, as the

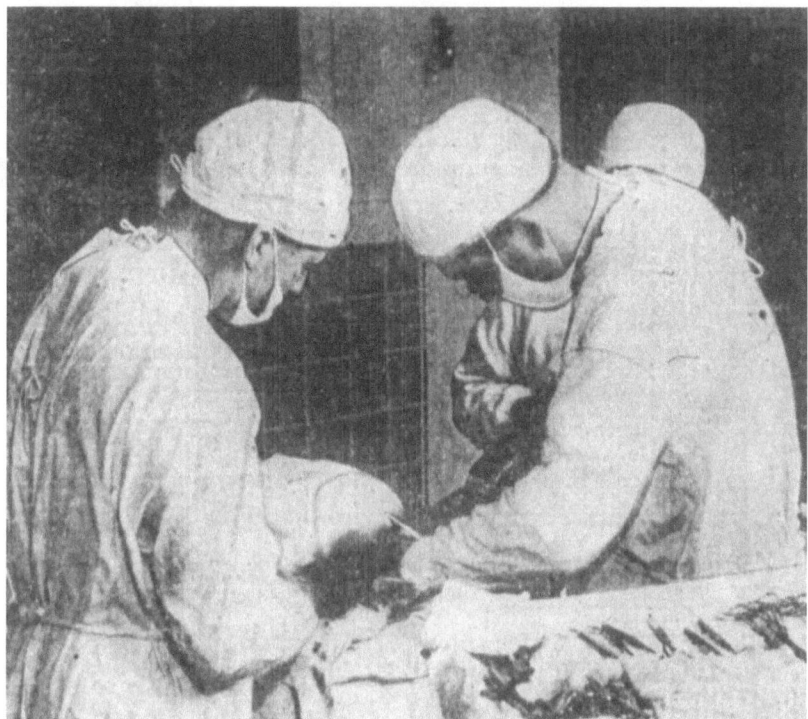

FIGURE 5.4. On October 25, 1931, the *Oakland Tribune* lauded community health meetings and the wonders that medicine could now accomplish. This photo appeared under the headline "Surgeons Perform Miracle of Science."

College had claimed in its cancer talks. The standard hospital and standard medicine were now nothing short of *spectacular*.

Perhaps the College thought the dire circumstances of the Depression provided a good context for talk of miracles: as though the miracles of medicine might translate into the personal miracles of desperate and destitute individuals in their everyday lives. This was, after all, the kind of connection between the personal and infrastructural that the College had spent years building.

But those at the College's helm in the early 1930s were also painfully aware that unless the College could latch onto a relevant medical issue once more, its position was vulnerable. The work that had taken up the majority of its time for over a decade—the imposition and marketing of hospital standardization—was perceived as essentially done. Medicine had moved on, and the College needed to, too.

Franklin Martin, the College's founder and still its director-general, had the answer. The new focus would be the fraught issue of health care costs. In response to a report from the Committee on the Costs of Medical Care, which raised concerns, among other things, about the costs of "supplying medical service to the community," Martin argued for the College's involvement, not so much to evaluate and examine the related issues but to proselytize the medical profession's point of view. With unusual candor, he opined that the success of its campaign for hospital standardization was the credential needed to confirm the American College of Surgeons as medicine's spokesperson in this arena too, just as surgical standardization had provided the necessary credential for hospital standardization. Someone needed to make insurance work, he said, and "we will do it just as we did . . . the hospital standardization movement." He continued:

> We did it two or three years before they realized what was going on. We quietly sent out agents and finally convinced the public that we were sincere and we finally convinced the surgeons that we were getting somewhere, and finally the whole medical profession realized the leadership in the American College of Surgeons in the several things it has attempted. [We] have succeeded beyond [our] fondest expectations. [We] will do the same with this.[67]

The talks of the early 1930s reflected new ambitions to get involved on this score. Robert Jolly, Baptist minister, hospital superintendent, and College evangelist, especially effortlessly shifted gears from standardization talk to educating the public on the question of health care costs. Jolly insisted that health costs were at the same time reasonable—people simply needed to save for their health as they would for a new car, he said—and the government's fault. The government's refusal to use voluntary hospitals for the care of veterans had deprived these hospitals of an income stream. And government bailouts of those hit hardest by the Depression created an unhealthy expectation for free care that threatened to further deplete the pocketbooks of medical professionals.[68] "It is a fact," agreed another commentator in Boston in 1934, "that people are getting in their minds that it is the duty of someone to take care of them" and, as consequence, were evading paying their bills.[69] Medical practitioners, these talks concluded, were left to pay the price. Quite in spite of Squier's glowing assessment of the medical marketplace, then, it looked like there *could* actually be too much health care, or at least that the profession was not quite as depression-proof as it had seemed.

But the College's commitment to this line of attack was never strong. Indeed, by the mid-1930s, it was actively advocating instead for a comprehensive overhaul of the payment system, emphasizing, as its commitment to standardization suggested it should, a rationalization of costs that would make health care uniformly affordable.[70]

In this, it never played as major a role as it had hoped. Martin died in 1935, perhaps taking some of the wind out of the effort's sails. In any event, over the next decade, the story of health care costs turned on the efforts of another organization, the AMA. It returned to center stage, deploying the same language the College had used in its effort to attach standard care to personal well-being, this time in the cause of preserving the profit-driven, privatized medical sector. This was the same medical sector that the College had sold to consumers as altruistic, unselfish to a fault, lifesaving, miraculous and so high-minded that it gave medical advice away for free. As it turned out, that medical advice was anything but free; it was, for its critics at least, merely the very successful sample product meant to induce the public to buy, buy, buy.

6

Monopoly

Let the big business men who would reorganize medical practice, the efficiency engineers who would make doctors the cogs of their governmental machines, give a little of their sixty horse power brains to a realization of the fact that Americans prefer to be human beings.—MORRIS FISHBEIN, "The Report on the Committee on the Costs of Medical Care," 1932

It was the autumn of 1938, and the members of the board of the Tampa Municipal Hospital were in a state of highest dudgeon. On October 17, they had learned through a press release that their hospital was being downgraded from its coveted position on the "approved" list of standardized hospitals of the American College of Surgeons to "provisional." Knowing that this sudden demotion would almost assuredly trigger a decline in business, and also insulted that they had not been directly and privately informed of this news by the College, the hospital board turned to the local paper to tell its side of the story. A fortnight later, the front page of the *Tampa Tribune* carried their angry message, alongside an article sympathetic to the hospital's situation. The two pieces ran under the headline, "Lid Off in Hospital Row."[1]

According to the hospital board, it had all started six months earlier with the customary drafting of the next year's hospital staff roster, which was to go into effect at the start of June. The main change from the previous year's list was the replacement of its superintendent with a roentgenologist (the precursor to the radiologist), one Dr. Sprinkle, who would hold both roles simultaneously. In part, this had been a strategic maneuver to settle a small controversy over X-ray fees. But there was also positive precedent: another roentgenologist, Dr. R. E. Baldwin, had held both roles simultaneously in 1932, with results that the board declared to have been "highly satisfactory."[2]

Dr. Sprinkle's rise to his dual role was accompanied by other minor new appointments, and as it had for many years, the hospital board also considered applications from physicians vying for the privilege of using the Tampa Municipal Hospital space to treat their own patients. As usual, the board members evaluated each candidate's qualifications and then passed on its list to the staff advisory committee for approval. This was given, and the new staff took up their posts on June 1.

Then came a sudden storm. Nine physicians who were not members of the county medical society had made their way onto the staff, and the staff physicians who were members wanted them out with immediate effect. "Despite the fact," the board members explained in their op-ed,

> that each physician appointed to the staff for [that] year was approved by the staff as then constituted, the [newly appointed] advisory committee of the staff protested to the board that physicians had been appointed to the staff who were not members of the Hillsborough County Medical society and that these men should be removed from the staff.[3]

In response to this membership protest, the board wrote to the three relevant hospital-certifying bodies to alert them to the changes that it had made. These were the American College of Surgeons (ACS), the relatively progressive American Hospital Association (AHA), and the veritable godfather of what was by then called "organized medicine," the American Medical Association (AMA). The AHA was apparently undisturbed by the board's changes and wrote back to the hospital board to say that as far as the AHA was concerned, "the Tampa hospital was an institutional member of the organization in good standing." The AMA answered that the hospital would remain on the list of approved hospitals to be published that August but warned that if the offending members of the staff were not removed by the time of its reaccreditation for 1939, that status would likely be withdrawn.[4]

The College was the least accommodating. Though the hospital board invited an ACS representative to travel to Tampa to reinspect the hospital and even offered to pay the expenses of this representative, the College declined. Instead, its office responded with an inventory of deficiencies derived from the board's own description of its changes. The most glaring shortcomings were those the hospital board members spent the bulk of their time addressing in their statement in the *Tampa Tribune*—namely, Dr. Sprinkle's dual role as roentgenologist-superintendent and the unacceptable presence of nonmembers of the local medical society on the hospital rolls for 1938.

Since the College did not send a new representative to survey the hospital in person, the board considered its approved status with the ACS to be safe in the meantime, as had been the case with the AMA. It came as a shock, then, when the news reached the board in mid-October that the ACS had rescinded its "approved" status. Finding themselves short a critical plaque on their wall of accreditation, the board members summarily fired Dr. Sprinkle as superintendent and hastily removed the nine offending staff members, informing the staff that the roster would, from that point onward, "be limited to members of organized medicine."[5]

This capitulation, the board members made clear, did not mean that they considered this the right thing to do. Hoping to impress on the Tampa public the injustice, not to mention the pettiness, of this turn of events, the board members took a great deal of care explaining the medical politics behind what they felt was their unfair censure. The board claimed the right to name its own staff and evaluate them on their "qualifications, ability and character"—attributes that had nothing to do with their attachment to a local medical society. That they had not been allowed to freely exercise this right, that they had been pressured by the local medical society and the AMA and actively punished by the College for appointing these nine nonmembers, amounted to obvious coercion.

Further, even as it caved to the College's demands, the board expressed the hope that its actions would catalyze a crisis by giving the nine ostracized nonmembers a clear path toward taking legal action against the local medical society, the AMA, the ACS, and anyone else who refused to acknowledge their right to practice. "The hospital board in informal discussions has sought to emphasize and make clear," the companion article explained, "that it is not attacking the professional standing of physicians and surgeons who will not be given staff appointments." Instead, it sought to highlight that this "law has been laid down by parent medical associations" like the AMA and the ACS—the same from whom the hospital is obliged to get "full approval for the hospital." Though organized medicine, as this bureaucratic club was known, had them over a barrel, the board retained the "full expectation that such compliance will be attacked in Florida courts by responsible doctors denied the right to practice their profession in a publicly-owned hospital."[6]

This recommendation of legal redress was acutely attuned to events taking place further north. In Washington, DC, just two weeks earlier, Assistant Attorney General of the United States Thurman Arnold had empaneled a grand jury to consider the question of whether the American Medical Association, along with the medical society of the District of Columbia and a dozen individual physicians, could be indicted under antitrust legislation for their actions in "restraint of trade" against the Group Health Association in Washington, DC. Quoting Arnold, the board's statement held that "organized medicine" could not "use organized power to advance, by economic pressure, coercion and boycott, the views of a particular group." Nor could they "use staff restrictions as a means of destroying the freedom of qualified physicians . . . to carry on their calling."[7]

As the board saw it, that was just what was happening right there in Tampa, as well as across the country.[8] More and more, certification requirements for hospitals, among their other more useful attributes, had become a convenient and powerful tool by which professional medical bodies could discipline medical practitioners and institutions acting in ways the associations considered injurious to their goals. In Tampa, the issue was contract work, with the hospital censure marking the boiling point of a long-simmering controversy between local medical societies and physicians in the community. The nine doctors struck from the roster were not just nonmembers of the county medical society. They had also committed the crime of having become salaried employees elsewhere, in breach of organized medicine's demand that physicians charge their patients exclusively in a "fee for service" arrangement. Although in this case the ACS stood out for its quick and drastic countermeasures, it would soon be matched and then overshadowed by the actions of the powerful AMA. Having achieved a new place in American life through its embrace and marketing of efficiency and standardization, medicine was now drawing on a different industrial force—monopoly—to consolidate its position.

This chapter explores how American medicine found new power and prospects in its role as a capitalist force, both leading up to and after the US government's successful prosecution of the AMA for violation of the Sherman Antitrust Act. For those who regard industrial efficiency as having laid the necessary groundwork for industrial capitalism, this might seem like a familiar story.[9] But just as elsewhere in medicine's history, efficiency's role in this story is harder to pin down. Indeed, for Arnold, the head of the antitrust division and prosecutor on the AMA case, efficiency lay on the opposite side of this equation: something like the antidote to the kind of bad behavior that built so many of the monopolies that, in turn, made capitalism run.

And it was not just those prosecuting organized medicine who held up efficiency as a principle in opposition to its work and aims. During this period, the AMA itself spearheaded a dramatic reorientation toward what had been so instrumental in elevating allopathic medicine above its competition. Now, efficiency would be equated with "socialism," an anti-American force that "tends to lower standards" because it "destroy[s] the incentive for professional advancement and professional achievement."[10] Further, efficiency was now antithetical to the good care uniquely found in the beneficial vagaries of the doctor-patient relationship, which only the fee-for-service model of reimbursement protected. As for the all-important standards of medicine that efficiency-minded reformers had worked to create, these were replaced by and deemed antithetical to a rubric of innovation and invention: characteristics better befitting the free market capitalism the AMA now sold itself as protecting.[11]

The discursive polarization of efficiency into the either/or of capitalist complicity that emerges out of this story is critical. It points to the larger picture of efficiency during the 1930s, when economists, political scientists, and journalists fought a war of ideas over the role that efficiency had played in the Depression. Depending on whom you asked and at what point in the Depression, efficiency seemed either the root cause of the economic crisis or its clear solution. The space it had once inhabited, somewhere in between these two poles, had become so narrow as to become nonexistent: in the quest for solutions to the catastrophe of the Great Depression, there was no room for—or interest in—any more expansive view of efficiency. This new polarization so totally obscured, both in rhetorical and real terms, the workings and characteristics of the preceding decades of efficiency that the fuller picture of its meaning and significance—as well as those of scientific management, Fordism, and Taylorism—would only become legible again when a revisionist history of labor rescued it from obscurity at the end of the twentieth century.[12]

This story of medical monopoly certainly helps flesh out how this larger polarization took place. But it also points to the specifics of the medical context and the making of a medical discourse that persists today. Though emphasis on the significance of the doctor-patient relationship had been a mainstay of AMA speeches and marketing well before the 1930s (not least as part of its attempts to maintain the fee-for-service structure implied by this relationship), it was in this period that the image of the doctor-patient relationship became firmly established as the preferred antithesis to efficiency and standardization. It heralded a new medical calculus with reconfigured equations. One held efficiency as equal to socialism, which in turn equaled ineffective and uncaring care. A second held up *inefficiency* as a core root value both of the doctor-patient relationship (in a fee-for-service model) *and* truly effective care.[13]

In this way, the AMA attempted—with a great degree of success—to recast American medicine, branding it as effective only when it was supremely inefficient (and, therefore, as costly as it needed to be). In doing so, it set the terms of debate still used in opposing nationalized forms of health care. That is, though not always explicitly called "socialized medicine," the various plans of nationalized or universal health care that have been proposed are nonetheless still commonly described as coming at the cost of innovation, progress, and individualized care—just as the AMA framed it almost a century ago. In this, the AMA broke with the preceding two decades of enthusiasm for standardization and efficiency as precisely the tools needed to create innovation, to foment the kind of democracy needed for the modern age, and to make space for the fullest expression of individuality. In one fell swoop, they both condemned the standardization efforts that had made medicine and rewrote medicine's early twentieth-century history.

So dominant was this view that the AMA also managed to re-create what we take as the essential components of good medical care. Though historians of medicine have been expansive in their analyses of how medicine has unfolded, the popular view persists that in order to understand medicine, we need to understand that its power stems from all of the qualities—the individualized attention, the explicit inefficiency of a healing relationship, the innovative personalized treatments—that hold up the doctor-patient relationship as the keystone of real and effective care.[14]

Group Practice

Common to histories of the AMA's monopoly prosecution is a description of organized medicine's heavy-handed response against what was called "group practice."[15] Though in previous decades the term had referenced the efficiency or "assembly line" style of doing medicine, since the late 1920s, group practice became a catchall descriptor for medical organizations that operated on a prepayment basis. This was not, then, the group practice of the Mayo Clinic, which maintained a fee-for-service billing arrangement even as it embraced an assembly-line service of medical care and a closed staff in the late 1910s. Nor was it exactly the group practice model of the Henry Ford Hospital, which also earned this moniker based on its assembly-line care system (though the comparison is closer here given the Fordist demand to set and prepublish flat fees and the outrage of the local medical society to this plan during the early 1920s).

It was this particular brand of group practice that went from being bad-mouthed to being actively and effectively opposed by a host of explicitly coercive measures in the 1920s. As the political scientist Oliver Garceau described in 1940, the change was abrupt. For decades from the late nineteenth to early twentieth century, he wrote, "many a big wig" physician ha[d] served a railroad without losing caste." So it was something remarkable when the East Baton Rouge Medical Society expelled a number of members for contract work at the "Stanacola Employees' Medical Association" in 1929.[16]

Hitherto a punishment meted out primarily for ethical abuses or egregious malpractice, expulsion quickly became a tool for policing institutional pricing mandates. By 1930, Garceau showed, the AMA was "discussing in earnest the possibilities of using this weapon to punish those exploring any method of payment for medical services that varied from the fee for service system." By 1931, it had started wielding this new billy club through the local medical societies. In that year, it threatened to expel the staff of the Trinity Hospital in Little Rock, Arkansas, who it accused of instituting a "voluntary group insurance plan." Rather than be forced out of the local society, the staff resigned en masse.[17]

A similar situation surrounded Dr. Michael Shadid, who began a group practice in 1931 under the auspices of the Oklahoma Farmer's Union in Elk City. Though his prepayment plan hospital was held up as a model for economical, efficient, and effective medical practice, it required the combined political power of the farmer's union and the support of Oklahoma governor "Alfalfa Bill" Murray to thwart efforts by the medical society to pressure the state licensing board into disbarring Shadid.[18] Indeed, as the story goes, the local medical society wielded so much influence that it was able to get many of the doctors that Shadid recruited to his practice drafted during the war, which threatened to "endanger the life of his organization."[19]

Then there were the so-called Milk Bottle Wars, which began as a protest of the Cattaraugus County Medical Society in New York against the successful installation of a county health "demonstration" that had been backed by the philanthropic Milbank Fund. Though health improvements related to the largely preventive health measures taken in Cattaraugus County demonstrated the effectiveness of the system, organized medicine, displeased by the supposed socialization of health care that the fund's involvement had precipitated, worked to derail the venture.

Their mechanism was to be Albert Milbank's stock portfolio. Milbank, president of the Milbank Fund, was also a major stockholder of the Borden Company, which sold milk products; indeed, it was from this stock that the Milbank Fund derived 45 percent of its capital.[20] Several local medical societies seized on this fact, organizing a boycott of Borden products in 1935 that spread across major US cities, ultimately putting such a dent in the Borden Company's bottom line that Milbank, it is said, was forced to capitulate. He fired the fund's executive secretary, John Kingsbury, for the crime of having successfully improved the health of the people of Cattaraugus County, and publicly recanted, declaring himself an opponent of "socialized capitalism" and "socialized individualism," echoing the terms that the societies had used to suggest that Milbank was threatening the sacred right of Americans to "free enterprise."[21]

This rhetorical division, between "free enterprise" as protected by the AMA and "socialized individualism" as its antithesis revealed the great distance that efficiency had traveled in medicine in just a short time. The AMA's "free enterprise" effort was now increasingly at odds with the principles of efficiency, which in turn had become synonymous with what the AMA had started to derogatively call "socialism." Those on the so-called socialist side embraced this new view of efficiency as well, fleshing out still further the terms of debate. One of the champions of medical efficiency from the 1910s and 1920s, Michael Davis, had begun to view the operative measure of efficiency neither in terms of the production of standards or systems nor in terms of how efficiency might make medicine effective or transparent. Instead, he worried over the distribution of medical care across the country.[22] Indeed, for both sides, efficiency began to explicitly and almost singularly signify concerns about how medical care would be distributed, how more equitable access might be achieved, and to what degree medicine might be folded into the larger purview of the state.

It was a discursive shift catalyzed to a great degree by the Great Depression, manifested in the specific calling out of the failings of mass production, but even more so in the political shifts that the Depression gave rise to. Now told in the terms of a political debate—so that the operative choice was *only* between capitalism and socialism or capitalism and fascism (or fascism and socialism, for that matter)—this rift also reflected the polarization of medical efficiency.[23] No longer descriptive of a broad range of interventions connected by a loose conglomeration of discernible qualities, and no longer representative of a large collection of individuals, loosely affiliated groups, hospitals, or professional organizations, the new language of medicine demanded a choice of allegiance. One was either for free enterprise or one was for socialism or even "sovietism," as the incendiary *Journal of the American Medical Association* and its editor Morris Fishbein condemned all the various enemies of the AMA.[24]

The reorientation along politico-economic lines continued. In 1934, the AMA's Bureau of Medical Economics published a document containing ten principles for the establishment of private health plans. One of the most important changes outlined therein was the AMA's bold refutation of "market free choice" in medicine and its replacement with a "guild free choice" model. Whereas market free choice had allowed for competition within medicine between different organizations and groups of physicians, especially on the basis of price, guild free choice effectively prohibited intra-professional competition by invoking the principle that, as the Bureau of Medical Economics described it, "'patients must have absolute freedom to choose a legally qualified doctor of medicine who will serve them from among all those qualified to practice.'"[25] Any medical payment plans that limited the number of physicians that a patient would be allowed to see—which prepayment plans did as a rule since they limited access to a certain group of providers—thus violated the AMA's transparent attempt to control pricing, thinly veiled as a protection of the free choice of patients to choose any doctor who would have them.[26]

In 1938, then, the Tampa Municipal Hospital found itself the latest point in a decade-long timeline of action against alternative medical pricing. The nine doctors struck from the roster were first attacked for not being members of the local medical society, but their chief sin—the one that had likely seen their dismissal from the medical society in the first place—was being employed in the prepayment group practice plans of the local Latin social clubs. Founded by immigrants for immigrants, these clubs were located mainly in the city's cigar-making Ybor City enclave. In exchange for weekly dues, which comprised about 5 percent of a member's salary, these clubs provided a package of social welfare, which included the comprehensive medical care that the physicians in question provided, an especially critical feature during the Depression.

Reformers were broadly sympathetic to these organizations. As the hospital administrator and medical efficiency enthusiast S. S. Goldwater put it early on, in 1915, "between the slip-shod service of the poorer kind of dispensary and the painstaking care of the conscientious lodge doctor, the choice easily lies with the latter."[27] Goldwater did not reference race in the context of these lodges, but he probably knew that in his native New York and around the country, lodge practice was filling the void of medical care not only for the nation's poor but also for immigrant and Black communities, especially in the South.[28]

It wasn't a perfect solution. For one thing, as Michael Davis noted in a 1937 examination of Black medical care in particular, lodge practice could only be as good—and, more importantly, as stable—as the membership that supported it. Medical practice at a small lodge, where the financial difficulties of only a few members would have a large financial impact, was less effective than at a large lodge, which had more financial resources to maintain steady services even when individual members suffered financial hardship.[29]

What made the Tampa lodge practices so successful was their popularity and size. El Centro Asturiano had already been a large and active club in Havana before its arrival in Tampa, where, from its founding, it was immediately five hundred members strong, growing from there by expanding its membership to other immigrant communities. Its main rival, El Centro Español, also grew in size over this period. Both were committed to health care as a rule, and both, in the first decade of the twentieth century, had enough funds to open their own hospitals.[30] And these hospitals were successful. Indeed, in the first decade after the founding of El Centro Asturiano's hospital in 1905, it stayed in the black. "The income from El Centro Asturiano's membership fees, canteen receipts, and social activities consistently exceeded expenses from the ... hospital."[31] Indeed, given the more general state of Tampa's municipal hospital over the first two decades of the twentieth century, it has been convincingly posited that the residents of Ybor City had the best health care in Tampa.[32]

Both their success and, more importantly, their explicit commitment to cooperative medical care put these organizations on the wrong side of the standardizing organizations of the day. In a set of coercive tactics that repeated themselves wherever this kind of group practice was found, the local medical society, with the devolved power of the AMA, attempted to shut down these prepayment practices, not by opposing them directly but by so constraining the careers of those physicians who might be involved in these reimbursement arrangements that they effectively could not practice. Stripping away the luxuries and protections that came with membership in the AMA was bad. But worse was the restriction that the threat of hospital disaccreditation placed on a blacklisted physician's ability to treat patients. Not all lodges came with their own hospitals, and not all lodge hospitals could do everything their counterparts could, especially as time went on. During the 1930s, those without the right to practice at a hospital were hardly doctors at all in the increasingly hospital-centric medical world that the ACS had especially worked to create.[33]

Monopoly

These events all came to a head in October 1938, just in time to add vigor to the Tampa hospital board's call for legal action. That month, a grand jury was empaneled in Washington to hear arguments in what would eventually be known as *The United States of America, Appellants, v. The American Medical Association, A Corporation; The Harris County Medical Society, An Association, et al., Appellees*. The case was finally resolved in 1943 when the AMA and Harris County Medical Society were found guilty and made to pay nominal fees, with the individual appellees exonerated.[34]

The particulars of this case, which led to an indictment and, ultimately, a guilty verdict, were not very different from what was happening elsewhere. In 1937, "2500 government employees, principally from the lower salary classes" had formed the Group Health Association, Inc. (GHA) "to provide prepaid medical care at a cost which the members could afford to pay."[35] The reaction of organized medicine to the GHA was more or less predictable, with the now customary deployment of expulsions and threats. The formation of the GHA was slowed further by a lawsuit filed on the part of the District Medical Society, which accused the GHA of "practicing medicine as a corporation" or, if not that, then being "engaged in the insurance business."[36] This lawsuit was dismissed, but the lengths to which the medical society had gone to stop the GHA suggested the specialness of the case. It not only involved federal employees but had also been organized in the first place with funds from a federal starter grant. In effect, it was a group health plan backed by the federal government—a partnership the AMA desperately wanted to dissolve.

The significance of this legal proceeding, the first of the antitrust lawsuits filed against the AMA and its various constituent parts, has often been described in terms of the health care politics of the late twentieth and early twenty-first century. That is, the lawsuit has been construed as the federal government's first and forceful foray into the construction of a national health insurance program, folded into Franklin Roosevelt's New Deal slate of social welfare reforms. Designed to expose and delegitimate the nefarious actions of the AMA, a successful prosecution or even a successful indictment of the AMA might have offered the mandate the government needed to enact change at the federal level.[37]

But as more legally minded scholarship has observed, the triggering situation for the prosecution of the AMA was more than *just* the federal government's potential designs on health care. The prosecution of the AMA was also steeped in the economic uncertainties of the Great Depression, which had resulted in the shifting fortunes of antitrust legislation.

Of course, the AMA's opposition to any model of reimbursement that was not on a fee-for-service basis was not new in the 1930s, as the vociferous opposition to the Fordist pricing policy of the Ford Hospital vividly demonstrated. But their tactics were emboldened by the shifting terrain of antitrust policies in the late 1920s and early 1930s, which had as their capstone the passage of the National Industrial Recovery Act (NIRA) in 1933. This legislation had to no small degree rolled back antitrust law on the principle that "self-regulation" would do more than "market competition" to stimulate the stalled economy.[38]

It was a prescription well suited to a popular diagnosis of the Depression's cause—namely, that the Depression was the result of a combination of overproduction and underconsumption. In 1933, an article titled "Dollars, Doctors, and Disease" appeared in *The Atlantic*, written by one of the primary proponents of this theory, the economist William Trufant Foster. He attempted to describe the logic, notably bundling medicine with other essentials, like food and housing, into his assessment:

> Why must so many thousands go hungry? Because we have produced too much corn and wheat, too many apples and potatoes, too much food of all kinds. Why must anybody suffer from cold? Because we have produced far too much coal and fuel oil, too much wool, too many woolen mills, too much clothing. Why must anybody live in shabby houses? Because we have surplus lumber, steel, copper, cement, hardware, and surplus carpenters, plumbers, painters, masons, architects, and contractors. . . . Precisely the same conditions now affect the medical profession. At least one hundred thousand persons in the United States sorely need hospital care to-day, but are not getting it. Why not? The answer seems to be that only two thirds of the beds in our private hospitals are in use, and the hospitals do not know what to do with their surplus capacity. . . . Many millions of men, women, and children suffer from other preventable diseases. Why is nothing done about that? The answer is that the science of preventive medicine has made marvelous advances in recent years, and tens of thousands of competent physicians are eager to use their new knowledge and their idle hours to save humanity from needless suffering.[39]

In making this case, Foster echoed what a lot of his contemporaries also believed: that large businesses were producing too much, driving prices too low, and in this way driving other firms out of business, with corresponding losses to the economy in the form of lost employment opportunity and reduced purchasing power.⁴⁰ The Ford Motor Company was, of course, one of the chief exemplars. Though Ford increased wages in response to the Depression—again, under the prevailing logic that higher wages increased purchasing power, which in turn would correct the problem of underconsumption—the company's position as the paragon of overproduction figured prominently.⁴¹ NIRA's solution to this problem was to allow cartelization within industries, such that each industry would "collude" to set the regulations of the industry as whole. This was explicitly the solution to the problem of large corporations like Ford, which so dominated the industry that their corporate regulations were effectively tantamount to those of the entire industry, advantageous to Ford but not necessarily to others. Cartelization was one answer, then, to the "ruinous competition" that Henry Ford and others of his ilk had created by their monopolization of the market.⁴²

To the AMA, this new path of cartelization seemed to indicate that the federal government was coming around to the point of view of professional organizations like itself and beginning to acknowledge its right to total control over the medical marketplace.⁴³ As Fishbein put it in 1935, the function of the NIRA seemed indeed to be "'closely analogous to those long conducted by professional associations and would seem to indicate that industry is finding it desirable to follow professional models rather than the reverse.'"⁴⁴ Drawing parallels from their situation to the industrial one, the AMA seemed to view "collusion among physicians through their medical societies" as not only "permissible" but fully and officially sanctioned by government policy. Instead of being the dominant Ford of the medical industry, they would be the cartel that would prevent the Fords from taking over.⁴⁵

But the pro-business legislative situation that had seemed to give the go-ahead to the AMA to pursue its new more heavy-handed enforcement practices was short-lived. NIRA was struck down by the Supreme Court in 1935.⁴⁶ By 1938, when the case's prosecutor Thurman Arnold took over the reins of the antitrust division at the Department of Justice, the legal landscape had changed completely. Instead of promoting cartels, the government was now primed to regulate monopolies, and the practices of the AMA had placed it squarely in Arnold's sights.⁴⁷

In a way, the guilty verdict was the least interesting thing about the United States of America versus the American Medical Association. For one thing, the Supreme Court declined to weigh in on a core question that the case turned on: whether medicine was a "profession," thus exempting the AMA from prosecution, or a trade, in which case it was fully subject to all antitrust legislation. This definitional problem was given new weight by the belief that NIRA had actively supported what looked like the application of professional mores in the industrial context. Attorneys for the AMA argued that, as a profession, medicine was not subject to the provisions of antitrust legislation—instead, this was an intraprofessional dispute outside the government's purview.[48] The district court agreed with this assessment, holding that the word *trade* did not include the "learned professions."[49] The appeals court, however, disagreed.

Hoping for a reversal, the AMA brought the case to the Supreme Court, which unhelpfully sidestepped all of this by noting that the Sherman Antitrust Act had used the far vaguer term "any person" in its discussion of those who might be acting in restraint of trade. Having determined that the GHA *was* engaged in trade by virtue of its prepayment plan business, the only real question was whether or not the actions of the AMA, as a group of "any persons," constituted its restraint.[50] Though the Supreme Court upheld the appeals court decision, its finding avoided any resolution on the question of the status of medicine, leaving open the question of how well antitrust legislation could ever control the actions of the profession of organized medicine.[51]

Though it left much still unresolved, the Supreme Court's verdict did cement a continued critical role for efficiency in these discussions. For Arnold, like Louis Brandeis before him, efficiency remained a key marker of the legitimacy of any business enterprise. As Brandeis had put it in a 1912 essay in *Collier's Weekly*, "Trusts, Efficiency, and the New Party," "no conspicuous American trust owes its existence to the desire for increased efficiency . . . on the contrary, the purpose of combining has often been to curb efficiency or even to preserve inefficiency, thus frustrating the natural law of survival of the fittest."[52]

Over the intervening years, and certainly during the first years of the Depression, efficiency had reentered discussions as a causal factor in the overproduction thesis. The Ford Motor Company was, of course, the poster child for both efficiency *and* what, by the early 1930s, looked to some as its resulting overproduction. The suggested correction—cartelization—thus emphasized something like the opposite of efficiency: an anticompetitive, actively encouraged intra-industrial collusion to stabilize prices.

Though Arnold broke from Brandeis on any sort of intrinsic relationship between bigness and (in)efficiency, he too maintained a faith in efficiency as an antidote both to corruption and to the woes of the Depression-era economy. If a corporation could acquire its size and power through efficiency, wrote Arnold in his various fulminations on the matter, it remained on the right side of the law. In this sense, efficiency had returned as something of the guarantor of a good and stable economy, insofar as it could bring the public the "savings of mass distribution and production."[53] On the other hand, if a corporation acquired its power through the "eliminat[ion] [of] competition by aggression or merger," this was a violation of antitrust law.[54] Efficiency's formerly expansive set of practices and meanings were now narrowed down to a simple dichotomy, and what Arnold considered to be the collusionist, coercive, and even "aggressive" practices of the AMA had placed the organization firmly on the side of monopoly.

Miraculous Medicine

All this placed the AMA in rather uncomfortable company. As he remarked privately, the AMA was made to seem a "predatory, antisocial monopoly."[55] But the further implications of this divide and the fleshing out of what each side offered came from the new discursive character of medicine as a lifesaving, miraculous good. As the community health meetings of the American College of Surgeons well document, the marketing of "standardized" health care had moved from selling the promise of standards themselves to solve and maintain health to hawking the promise of both personal attention and miracle cures.

As the 1930s rolled in, the ACS no longer saw a need for its community health meetings. Having sold the public so successfully, it thought, on the promise of the standardized hospital, there was nothing left to do but to turn toward the thorny problem its success had created: how to provide health care for this public now (purportedly) completely sold on medical care at a moment when few had the financial resources to actually acquire it.[56]

Medicine's new discursive position was certainly evident in the landmark 1932 final report of the Committee on the Costs of Medical Care (CCMC), which originally convened in 1928 to investigate the growing crisis of medical economics. Though the report drew the ire of organized medicine, whose representatives on the committee responded with a "minority report" of their own, there was no difference of opinion on how critically important, miraculous, and lifesaving medicine was. In words entirely befitting the College's itinerant community health preachers, the CCMC majority report lauded the progress of medicine over the preceding decades. "Within the span of a single lifetime," it dramatically began,

> the widespread utilization of anesthesia, aseptic surgery, bacteriology, physiology and radiography has revolutionized the practice of medicine. Even during the last decade, medicine's advance in the unending warfare against sickness is little short of miraculous. Physicians and other men of science have displayed an unparalleled generosity in making available

to their colleagues and thus to mankind the results of their research and inventive genius.[57]

With such heady rhetoric, the committee expressed the debt that society now owed to medicine in a way that would have shocked physicians just a decade earlier. The "inventive genius" and "unparalleled generosity" of physicians and other researchers, the "miraculous" progress of medicine that seemed so near and obvious in 1932, was a world away prior to even the mid-1920s.[58] The College's decision to certify surgeons and standardize hospitals in the late 1910s was, after all, driven not by medicine's miraculous qualities but by its embarrassing reality: practitioners and hospitals so uniformly shoddy that, especially in the case of hospitals, a bare minimum of improvements was the only practical, implementable program. That these hospitals were so terrible that small shifts actually did make a big difference is also testament to the fact that medicine in the early 1920s was hardly the panacea that commentators in the 1930s conjured up.

Though they did not fundamentally subvert this view of medicine's miraculousness, some critics called out this view at least on grounds that it was not miraculous everywhere. As Hugh Cabot, one of the most outspoken physician voices against the activities of the AMA, put it at the National Health Conference in 1938, however good medicine might be in some places, there remained "very large areas in this country where the practice of medicine as at present carried on is medieval."[59]

In fact, though politicians, public intellectuals, physicians, philanthropic organizations, and the other agents that guided public discussion of medicine in the 1930s agreed that medicine was a crucial public resource, there existed a still sizable portion of the population that had not yet been "standardized," as the American College of Surgeons would have put it. These citizens not only did not have access to the "standardized" hospitals that the College had been selling, but they also had not automatically embraced the College's paired claims that medical service was required for any and all body ailments and that this service must exclusively come from the hands of allopathic practitioners.

Of course, there were still lodge practices, even if they were less popular in the 1930s than in the decade before. For many, they remained a critical alternative to mainstream health care, especially since rampant racism remained an essential element of health care across the board.[60] There was also still a strong market for patent medicines. Documents like the CCMC majority report point out with concern that spending on "secret formular medicines," obtainable over the counter, still comprised 10 percent of the total of all per annum spending on medical services and commodities in the early 1930s, to the tune of a healthy $360 million.[61] An additional $125 million was spent on visits to non-allopathic practitioners: an impressive figure given the fact that these "cult" practitioners comprised an ever-dwindling portion of the medical population.[62] But despite these and other quibbles with the breadth and scope of allopathic practice, in the public arena, the narrative of miraculous modern medicine took firm hold, framing the debate.

Medicine's success had significant drawbacks. One of the critical implications of the acceptance of the view that medicine was miraculous and lifesaving was that it became everybody's business: a service so successful for a good so essential—health—that it ought to be distributed equally to all. And though, on the one hand, organized medicine deserved credit for this achievement, on the other hand, in the words of the pioneering medical historian Richard Shryock, it had so effectively "transform[ed] indifference into a growing public demand for medical service" that it found itself not celebrated for having invented it but vilified for refusing to share this essential resource equitably.[63]

Indeed, the "miraculous" medicine the CCMC report invoked by way of introduction was not the prelude to a prayer of thanksgiving for "organized medicine." It instead preceded an argument for removing medicine from the control of what had been increasingly described as its monopolistic organizers. Such a precious resource, the committee's work implied, could no longer be *just* a commodity left to the whims of a single group. Something so essential had to be given as a right to all citizens. As Foster's inclusion of medicine in and among the other items of overproduction attested, medicine had achieved a vaunted position: like housing and food, it was considered an essential. Though in part reflecting what many believed was the real-time value of health care, it was also a move with potentially considerable political heft, since it freed medicine up to be considered, like food and housing, within the burgeoning rubric of Roosevelt's New Deal legislation.

Critiques of medicine accepted the renowned historian of medicine Henry Sigerist's pithy description of this situation, when he described it as one in which the "technology of medicine had outrun its sociology."[64] The miracles and inventive genius—that was the technology. But its sociology, the now inappropriately monopolistic behavior of organized medicine, was no longer deemed the proper modern counterpart. In this way, medicine was drawn not only into the Depression era discourse of overproduction, but it was also given a makeover, transforming into an issue that fitted the polarized political language of socialism and capitalism, left and right, or, in more strictly medical terms, a socialized or even nationalized system of health care versus a capitalist, free market, private, for-profit system. It is a discourse that still defines the debate about health care systems today.

These new terms of debate were both created and bolstered by a new generation of muckrakers, now squarely viewed as on the political left. James Rorty (father of acclaimed philosopher Richard Rorty), who had a dalliance with communism a few years earlier, applied his zeal to the story of "organized medicine" in his 1939 *American Medicine Mobilizes*. Already well known for his anti-capitalist excoriation of the advertising industry, *Our Master's Voice*, Rorty had established himself as something of a political radical, working explicitly in the manner of (and drawing explicitly from) his near contemporary Thorstein Veblen. Indeed, his critique of advertising had centered on its role as capitalism's ideological and economic handmaiden.[65] His critique of medicine did much the same, setting medicine's table as polarized into two distinctive groups: those who were dedicated to the "conservative" agenda of "so-called organized medicine" and "an assortment of liberal doctors, social workers, trade unionists, public health officials, and others" whose attempts to modernize medicine and to bring it to the people were constantly being thwarted by medicine's capitalist tendencies.[66]

Though Rorty told the story of the AMA quite ably, fair and balanced he was not. After reading his work, readers were likely left with the same political or ideological convictions they had brought to it. Rather than win over the unconverted, Rorty's purpose instead seemed to be to write medicine into a developing script of anti-capitalism.

Another prominent critic was the political scientist Oliver Garceau. Though less hardline than Rorty and less propagandistic (according to reviewers), Garceau too laid out the case against the AMA in explicit detail, making it clear to readers that the responsibility for the problematic status of medicine lay at the feet of the AMA.[67]

Indeed, the news was everywhere.[68] On the eve of its indictment in 1938, a fairly scathing critique of the AMA appeared in the business-friendly *Fortune* magazine, which tied the AMA's problematic rise all the way back to its apparently innocuous decision, in 1881, to create a weekly journal. It did so, the article suggested, in order to facilitate raising funds for its activities: the selfsame that made possible its power acquisition process. The AMA "calculated," the *Fortune* article put it, "that the *Journal* distributed gratis to 25,000 members would cost $8,000 per year, but this would be offset by $12,500 in annual dues and by an estimated $5,800 in advertising revenues."[69] This financial gamble paid off, the article concluded. Not only did the journal turn a profit in its first years, allowing the AMA to pursue its standardizing agenda, but it kept the AMA comfortably in the black during the bleak years of the Depression. Indeed, in 1939, the AMA journal's gross profits were a whopping $1.65 million.[70]

As this article saw it, the *Journal of the American Medical Association* was something of a smoking gun. For unlike its well-respected contemporary the *Boston Medical and Surgical Journal* (better known since 1928 as the *New England Journal of Medicine*), which had been conceived of as a vehicle for the sharing of health care knowledge and experience, the AMA's journal was created to distribute its propaganda. Against this backdrop of other journals that were genuinely contributing to medical knowledge, the AMA's journal looked suspicious indeed.

According to another prominent critic, Bertram Bernheim, the AMA's main preoccupation was telling physicians who had little interest in things outside the specifics of medical practice who they were and what they stood for.[71]

The editors of the *Journal of the American Medical Association* certainly had a knack for filling it with simple messages, endlessly repeated. The *Journal* "believes strongly in the power of repetition," Garceau wrote, and though it sometimes did "add a little new frill to its supply of mythology," it never strayed from its central themes, but rather "repeats the entire preceding structure" of that mythology with each successive issue.[72] The *Journal* staff was also always happy to help the local medical societies fill their own journals with content. Local medical journals got their issues out, and the AMA found yet another venue to recycle and redeploy its messaging. Over time, Garceau noted, the AMA developed around the *Journal* an ever-broadening array of marketing materials. A "clipping bureau and a package service" were joined over the years by the pamphlets, booklets, posters, radio addresses, and outlines of lectures that stood at the ready for deployment to the local fronts by the 1930s. This was an apparatus that helped disseminate the AMA's views and was particularly effective once organized medicine came under attack, effectively heading off controversy in situ before it had the chance to develop nationally.[73]

These attacks on the *Journal* helped clarify to audiences of the 1930s who the relevant actors in "organized medicine" actually were. Though the term was typically used to refer to the body of medical practitioners who stood behind the AMA and the other major medical organizations of the day, its critics also wrote about the pharmaceutical companies, medical appliance businesses, and other concerns whose advertising dollars had made the *Journal* a financial success.[74] At one point, Rorty singled out a "lengthy chapter on the promotion of a well-known brand of cigarettes" that had been "obviously dragged in for the sensation it might create."[75]

The Doctor-Patient Relationship

In response to assertions of this kind, the AMA was left with the difficult challenge of inventing practically out of whole cloth a new justification for itself that, without backing away from medicine's indispensability, also did not admit that medicine was an essential service that a state owed to its citizens. At the same time, it needed to position itself as not so big that it posed a threat to the state, but also big enough to handle all aspects of health provision.

Its choices here, in its self-presentation, shifted the significance of medical efficiency profoundly. For what had made medicine so successful over the preceding decade—such that it had enjoyed a stellar reputation over that period—had been its embrace of medical efficiency not just for the systematization, rationalization, and standardization that this introduced but also for the hammering out of these principles in the ever-present context of efficiency's complex relationship to populism, democracy, and egalitarianism. To accept in place of this a reductive iteration of efficiency as antagonistic to capitalism was to acknowledge the end of that era's modernist way of doing medicine altogether.

Casting off the mantle of standardization and rationalization that had become so essential to medicine's modernization in the first place, Fishbein offered a new language to describe the medicine of a new era, which set not only free enterprise and capitalism against socialism but also effective care against efficient care. Painting a portrait of medical practitioners as taken by surprise by the incursion of socialist medicine, he described them as instead so focused on "their daily and nightly task of preventing disease, healing the sick and ministering to the afflicted" that they had "given scant attention and but little of their time to a consideration of the way in which their work was being invaded by the octopus of big business." But now that they had been alerted to the desires of big business to "organiz[e] and standardiz[e]" the country's way into health, they were ready to defend against an intrusion that, Fishbein claimed, would make both doctors and patients "cogs of their governmental machines." Physicians, he insisted, could not allow this to happen. Moreover, he suggested that the American people should not—would not—allow it to happen, either. Capturing an increasingly important rhetorical thread of contemporary debates about the purported drawbacks of efficiency, as these were being manifested especially in the context of the perceived overreach of New Deal big government, Fishbein made the explosive pronouncement that since "Americans prefer to be human beings," they should remain capitalists and thus reject the efficient, socialized, mass-produced medicine overtaking the country.[76]

Though brimming with irony, this new twist on efficiency stuck—and not only in medicine. Foreshadowing the fate of efficiency in our own contemporary world, views on the utility and significance of industrial efficiency were changing. By the 1970s, it would become commonplace to think that industrial efficiency provided the "quintessential form of managerial control" needed to achieve capitalism in the first decades of the twentieth century in the first place.[77] Any more nuanced view of efficiency had fallen victim to the Great Depression and its various attempted repairs.

Worthy of note was the AMA's brandishing of efficiency as both the manifestation of big business, with its tendencies toward monopoly, and as a socialist entity, with its tendency toward big government.[78] Indeed, in the same article where Fishbein lauded the purity and altruism of medical practitioners and lambasted the big business "octopus" that threatened the field, he suggested alternately that the specter of government intrusion into medical business might instead be "sovietist": distinctly dangerous to the real democratic, free market values that medicine had always so valiantly upheld.[79] By 1938, those lobbying for more equitable medical care through the busting of medicine's monopoly had been reduced in the discourse to either quacks or communists who threatened to steal patients from mainstream medicine by offering them a dangerous alternative to fee-for-service compensation arrangements.

The AMA's rather disjointed efforts at deflecting intrusions into its own monopoly—labeling its enemies variously as anticompetitive, socialist, technocratic, or dangerous quacks—were surprisingly successful. But far and away the most resonant of the AMA's claims about medicine was its insistence that government intrusion (or intrusion of any other kind, for that matter) into health care would deeply affect the precious and personal relationship between doctor and patient that was and always had been medicine's hallmark. That this hallmark of medical practice bore a distinctive link to capitalism, even if just by the AMA's rejection of other political affiliations, created the strange merry-go-round of discourse that accompanies health care today. Indeed, this effective but deeply misleading piece of rhetoric remains a part of the chorus of protests that are still launched at the possibility of a federalized health insurance program: that medicine and health are deeply personal services, such that if a patient is to be treated as a human being, they cannot be subjected to a health care intermediary who will transform the patient into a "standardized machine."[80]

Early on, Fishbein doubled down on this image of medical practitioners who were uniformly and personally invested in each and every patient, invoking the utterly unsubstantiated statistic that "more than 80 per cent of all the ailments for which people seek medical aid can be treated most cheaply and most satisfactorily by a family physician with what he can carry in a handbag."[81] Though at odds with what the AMA had claimed about the specialness and technological prowess of the modern physician, this claim caught on, appearing, among other places, in the AMA's marketing rebuttals of the findings of the CCMC majority report. Indeed, the National Physicians' Committee, formed in the wake of the antitrust lawsuit, had the explicit intention of using it to "flood all channels of propaganda—the daily, weekly, and trade papers; the magazines; the radio; public meetings and meetings of any other sympathetic groups."[82] That it also directly contradicted the original goals of medicine's standardization seemed utterly irrelevant. Indeed, the image the phrase conjured up, of the family physician offering personal care to a trusting patient, ultimately provided the impetus for the AMA's later campaign against a compulsory health insurance program in the 1950s.[83]

The death stroke—at least at that time—for a comprehensive federal health program in the United States came in the form of a painting. *The Doctor* had been produced in 1891 by the British artist Luke Fildes and featured a practitioner making a home visit. He sits vigil, leaning over a young patient, chin on fist. They are joined in the rather dilapidated lodging by the mother, her head buried in her arm at a table, with her husband's hand stoically placed on her back. Pressed into service to protect organized medicine from legislative onslaught in 1951, the image was accompanied by language that drove home the point that this precious personal relationship between the family physician and his young charge would be destroyed by efficiency. It was a Victorian social fantasy now rechristened as the American way (figure 6.1). So critical had this idealized personal relationship become to salvaging organized medicine's control over the monopoly it had built that it willingly sacrificed, for a time at least, the hard-won image of an efficient and thereby effective expert. The efficiency that had been essential to drumming up business in the 1910s had now been replaced by a practiced inefficiency of care. Whether effective or not, this was a doctor who would at least sit with you through the night.

This was a disingenuous defense, and critics who were also physicians knew it. Cabot immediately pounced: "It is difficult to understand ... these protests," he snapped in the *New York Times*, "since the only patients concerned [in the effort to extend medical access] were the very ones who rarely secure personal contracts under the traditional system of practice."[84] For those who had no doctor, the problem of how close the relationship might be between patient and doctor was simply irrelevant.

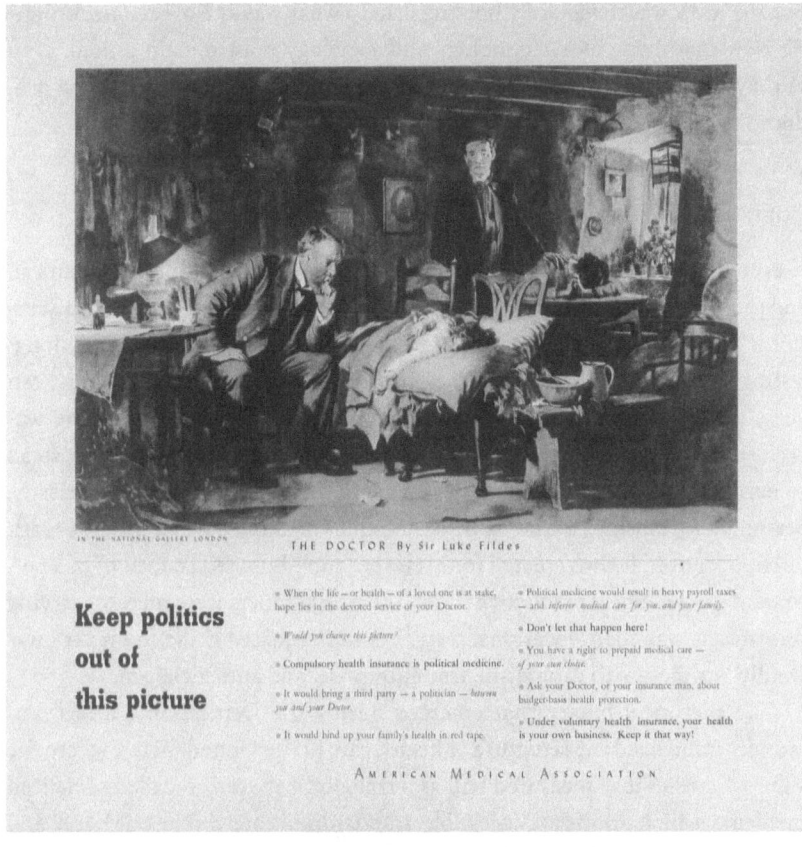

FIGURE 6.1. Luke Fildes's 1891 painting *The Doctor* became a mainstay of AMA marketing over the 1950s. Image courtesy of Yale University Library, Manuscript and Archives, New Haven, Connecticut.

The physician James Means, in his 1938 presidential address to the American College of Physicians, had another bone to pick, pointing out that the maintenance of the "sacrosanct doctor-patient relationship" would not be eroded but improved by the presence of a third party. "I submit," he said,

> that having a third party determine the size of, and even collect, the fee from the patient for the doctor is not only not an intrusion into the holy doctor-patient relationship but actually increases the likelihood of the patient's receiving from the doctor the best and wisest treatment the doctor is capable of giving.[85]

But the AMA was unyielding, holding firm to what was by now an anachronistic view that medicine's technology and sociology must remain united, even as they cast off the standardization and mass-production ethos that had produced this ideology in the first place.

Conclusion

If ever there was an archetypal image of the AMA as a ruthless, tyrannical, and problematically monopolistic operation, it was manifested in these discussions. The rhetoric itself has proved to be both effective and incredibly long-lasting. Even in the 1930s, with the chaotic medical marketplace of just ten years earlier still fresh in the public's memory, the history of medicine was actively being rewritten not to gloss its immediate industrial past but instead to jump backward first to Victorian England, then all the way to the priestly, personal relationships of the "time of Asclepius or those written into the Oath of Hippocrates." It thus created for itself the "time-honored tradition" of a personal, caring medical practice that medical practitioners were merely carrying forward, as was their vocational duty.[86] And it equated these, however awkwardly at times, with capitalism, free enterprise, and anti-socialism.

The rhetorical binary that emerged during the Depression era has profoundly influenced the structure of health care in the United States, where the value of medicine is measured still as a trade-off between so-called socialized medicine, which prioritizes accessible, standardized care, on the one hand, and the capitalist model of medicine, which emphasizes the care and personal attention of a doctor-patient relationship (at least for those who can afford it), on the other. Even though studies of European national contexts demonstrate that access is not a sure panacea, and though we know from our own experience that efficiency and compassionate care are not necessary contradictions, this binary remains firmly entrenched.

In the more prosaic terms of this book, however, the AMA and its efforts in the Depression era effectively ended the distinctively "modern" era of medicine that efficiency had built over the first decades of the twentieth century. It also ushered in a new narrative for itself in which allopathic medicine's superior "technology," as Sigerist put it, had been the ultimate deciding factor in raising allopathy above all other medical sects and where its dedication to the doctor-patient relationship essentially nullified calls to make health a social good. Although hardly an accurate historical rendering, the narrative has stuck.

Afterword

In the opening pages of his foundational 1972 text, *Effectiveness and Efficiency*, the physician Archie Cochrane traced the point of origin for his articulation of evidence-based medicine to his miserable experience as a World War II prisoner of war. One of the few POWs in the camp with any medical training, Cochrane had been charged with the impossible task of caring for the ill and dispensing the meager medical supplies on hand. "Under the best conditions," he wrote,

> one would have expected an appreciable mortality; there in the *Dulag* I expected hundreds to die of diphtheria alone in the absence of specific therapy. In point of fact there were only four deaths, of which three were due to gunshot wounds inflicted by the Germans. This excellent result had, of course, nothing to do with the therapy they received or my clinical skill. It demonstrated, on the other hand, very clearly the relative unimportance of therapy in comparison with the recuperative power of the human body. On one occasion . . . I asked the German *Stabsarzt* for more doctors to help me cope with these fantastic problems. He replied: "Nein! Ärtzte sind überflüssig!" ("No! Doctors are superfluous.") I was furious and even wrote a poem about it; later I wondered if he was wise or cruel; he was certainly right.[1]

This was not just an ocean but worlds away from the story of miraculous technology and treatment that the American Medical Association (AMA) had begun telling about medicine just a few decades earlier. Indeed, Cochrane found little to celebrate in his role as senior (because only) medical officer at the Salonika POW camp. Far more nihilistically, he turned to the double-blind trials that would become the hallmark of evidence-based medicine, with a logic that would have been intimately familiar to efficiency-minded medical practitioners of the 1910s and 1920s: the only way to make medicine effective—given its intrinsic "superfluity"—was to make it maximally efficient.

Cochrane's deployment of efficiency was twofold. He thought, as did some of his forebears in the early twentieth century, that the reentry of efficiency into medicine would curb the worst excesses of the profession, first by obligating tests of the effectiveness of any therapy or treatment before its widespread dissemination and then by forcing accountability and transparency back onto medical practitioners and their practices. One of the most sensational of Cochrane's early findings in this vein was, as summed up by one rather skeptical Canadian cardiologist, that "heart attack victims may actually be better off at home in bed instead of receiving the most scientifically advanced care in a hospital coronary care unit (CCU)."[2] Cochrane famously teased this finding to his colleagues, first showing them a table that suggested that the opposite was true: that CCU outcomes were far better than those at home. As he noted years later, their reply was one of horror: "Archie, that trial is unethical, it must be stopped at once!" Yet, when he, with feigned remorse, "showed them the correct table, with fewer deaths at home, and said, didn't they think it would be unethical to continue with coronary care units," they demurred, angry at the deception, but perhaps angrier still at the table's insinuation that the "most scientifically advanced care" was not obviously also the most effective care.[3]

Right down to his incendiary delivery and dramatic flair, Cochrane matched the brand of efficiency that the early twentieth-century surgeon, efficiency expert, and consummate provocateur Ernest Amory Codman had pursued in his own time. And Cochrane was not alone in seeing in efficiency a solution to what was essentially the same situation that Codman had worked against a half-century before—unmeasured outcomes, ineffective care, and arrogant colleagues. In the United States, Cochrane's contemporaries and fellow reformers were calling for change and indeed invoking Codman's name as the efficiency prophet that medicine had forgotten. The pages of medical journals were hosting the stuff of séances:

> I intend to summon from a shadowy past someone who should have been recognized always as a towering figure in the history of our field. It is Ernest Amory Codman whom I invoke. . . . I hope to celebrate the man, making amends, in my small way, for the neglect he has so long unjustly suffered.[4]

It was a prayer into the past that found Codman speaking right back. Having been "neglected" by his colleagues, as he put it in his wildly entertaining autobiographical preface to his study of the shoulder (that was also itself a paean to efficiency), he despaired that "honors, except those I have thrust on myself, are conspicuously absent from my chart." Nevertheless, he had high hopes for the future. "I am able to enjoy the hypothesis," he wrote, "that I may receive some from a more receptive generation."[5] Never mind that his published work on the shoulder, minus its excoriations of the medical field, was met with great appreciation in its time. Codman's message of reform was finding apostles amid this later "more receptive generation" just as he had foretold.

The period starting in the early 1970s was indeed a moment of reflective skepticism for some in medicine. One prominent view was that medicine had not actually been effective until the 1930s (and only questionably then). As Cochrane's colleague Thomas McKeown famously put it, it was not vaccination or other medical interventions but rather improvements in sanitation, agriculture, and nutrition that had so successfully turned the tide of infectious disease over the previous two centuries.[6] This was not a completely new notion—McKeown's work challenging the relationship between medical intervention and the reduction or amelioration of disease built on that of the immunologist Thomas Magill, whom he loved to quote. As Magill had put it when describing a chart depicting pneumonia rates in New York State over the past several decades:

> If we are disposed to be critical, we shall note that the steep downward trend in the pneumonia death-rate began to taper off in the early 1940's and that during the past few years the curve has followed a more or less horizontal course. It is of considerable interest that the initiation of that course of events coincided with the introduction of the antibiotics, and that the decline in death-rate essentially ceased as these agents became more and more universally employed. Are we to infer that those valuable agents have worsened the situation? I think not. It would seem to be a more logical conclusion that during recent years, quite regardless of our therapeutic efforts, a state of relative equilibrium has established itself between the microbes and the ever-varying state of the immunological constitution of the herd.[7]

Even as McKeown worked to popularize the sense that most things in health happened "quite regardless of . . . therapeutic effort," others were at work on their own takes. There was the radical priest Ivan Illich, who professed to "emphatically . . . not care about health," while calling out medicine as an autocratic, monopolistic entity representing the worst of capitalism. Medicine was, he said, merely a "prolific bureaucratic program based on the denial of each man's need to deal with pain, sickness, and death" that was characteristic of the "capital-intensive commodity production" essential to modernity.[8] In his view, the problem was less that medicine didn't work, it was that medicine's entire claim to effectiveness rested on little more than the power it had been able to acquire by its own self-aggrandizing claims of being so "scientifically advanced" that the question of its effectiveness was presented as asked and answered.

Buttressing this narrative were scholars of the "new social history of medicine" like Susan Reverby, David Rosner, and Charles Rosenberg, and their sociologist peers, like Nicholas Jewson, Eliot Freidson, and Paul Starr. Together they reframed medicine's history to accommodate the view that something other than scientific advancement—something that allowed it to make itself legible in capitalist terms—was medicine's modus operandi in the early twentieth century. This something was professionalization, which fit the bill of explaining how the establishment had become so powerful without commensurate advances in effectiveness.[9]

Some, like the inimitable E. Richard Brown, took an even darker view. In his study of the rather incestuous relationships between the Carnegie and Rockefeller foundations and the AMA and other medical professional organizations, he showed exactly how embedded and intersecting in the capitalist world "organized medicine" really was.[10] It was a classic paradigm shift. By the end of the decade, the new social historians of medicine had created an impressive body of literature that gave evidence to what many were feeling: that medicine's history was not the triumphant story of scientific progress and great men doing great things that it had told for itself; rather, it was a socially embedded narrative about capitalism, with medicine but one more convenient vessel for capitalism to fill up.[11]

These were the circumstances that made efficiency seem such a welcome reformist addition at the end of the twentieth century, with its promise to call everyone into line by forcing on them the presumptively objective appraisal—the "scientific," classificatory appraisal, as its early-century proponents would have insisted—that efficiency could provide. But just as in other areas of historical inquiry, efficiency was also and simultaneously explicitly tied to capitalism by the renaissance of Taylorism and Fordism as both capitalism's catalyst and its on-the-ground iterations. And in the political arena, efficiency retained the branding that the AMA had given it during the 1930s, as the socialist solution that would, as Sarah Palin put it in 2009, lead ineluctably to things like "death panels," where the value of a life would be calculated according to a person's "level of productivity" in society.[12]

Clearly, efficiency never lost its mojo. It is perhaps unsurprising that its trajectory should be so recursive and cacophonous and read in so many contradictory ways across such a long period.[13] Also unsurprising is that it should still be threading its willy-nilly way through the warp and weft of capitalism. After all, it was from its origin a contested value, with roots and goals in both democracy and autocracy simultaneously. And for all that, it was also a good barometer for the world that it occupied, feeling its way along and defining and redefining a set of conceptual truths about how the United States functioned and what it stood for as time progressed.

What is surprising, however, is how much the larger, longer history of efficiency (as medicine's modernizing handmaiden) has obscured a clearer view of what medicine is, what it actually does, and how it really functions. One way that efficiency suggests we might parse modern medicine and its history is as an information technology system. Though he was perhaps not intending to make a grand epistemological point, the computer scientist and physician Edward Shortliffe pithily suggested this view back in the 1990s, when he wrote that we might reasonably view "the practice of medicine [as] inherently an information management task."[14] That certainly would fit the bill for many of efficiency's protagonists who, like Cochrane and Codman before him, took the position that without a well-structured information management system, the practice of medicine was just a mixed bag of questionable diagnoses and dubious treatments—with a drop of elitism for good measure.

The lessons of this view of medicine certainly remain capitalism-adjacent. Understanding the practice of medicine as an information management system turns attention toward the question of *whose* information and to what end. Indeed, medical information was and remains only as representative as one makes it. For all the talk about egalitarianism, democracy, and social plasticity, efficiency only ever made medicine for the "great silent majority" to whom the American College of Surgeons peddled its "standardized" medical wares. This was the same silent majority that embraced Prohibition, bemoaned jazz, and voted the bland conservative Calvin Coolidge into office. Medicine in the 1920s was marketed to and indeed made for them, both explicitly, as an untapped medical market, and implicitly, as those whose ailments and medical wants shaped the production of medical knowledge.

As Flexner's own segregationist approach to the Black medical schools makes clear, the common problem of efficiency stemmed not from its ideological designs but from the application of that ideology to the real world, which was full of those who stood so far outside the silent majority as to find themselves utterly unrepresented in the information qua medical system that resulted. That the resulting system prioritized the whiteness and maleness of this silent majority is quite obviously still the case. And though the American College of Surgeons ended up selling standards as fundamentally personal, the standards it created were not even one-size-fits-all for those in its advertising demographic. That has been a harder lesson for the public to learn. But anyone who has read about difficult- or impossible-to-diagnose mystery illnesses in Lisa Sanders's *New York Times* "Diagnosis" column, or has been misdiagnosed or had their own illness not taken seriously—indeed, anyone who read the words of Allen Roses, the worldwide vice president of genetics at the pharmaceutical behemoth GlaxoSmithKline, who in 2003 confessed that from the ubiquitous Tylenol to the chemotherapeutic concoctions of cancer treatment, the "drugs don't work" in a lot of cases and certainly not in exactly the same way in any two people—will recognize that standard medicine only works in a standard way for a standard person, who unfortunately does not exist.[15] Such is the paradox that underlies "personalized" or "precision" medicine, which is understandably misunderstood to be both personal and precise. And such is the fallacy, too, that underlies the basic supposition of our contemporary mainstream medical models—namely, that either access alone or the doctor-patient relationship alone will be enough to make medicine truly inclusive.

Although this is by no means a new way to parse medicine, the history of efficiency offers a shifted perspective from which to pursue it. These ill effects were not simply the result of a "technology that had outrun its sociology" or the result of a project that was epistemologically pure but tainted by a wrong capitalist turn. Instead, they are as fundamentally intrinsic to modern medicine as they are to modernity more broadly. If we want to remake medicine as an inclusive and democratic entity, this logic suggests, then we may need to start again from scratch.

Fortunately, efficiency can also give us some inspiration as to how this might be done—not in practical terms, perhaps, but in ideological ones. We have generally dismissed this ideological bent toward democracy as a sign of efficiency's false consciousness. But medical efficiency (like efficiency more generally) emerged from an early twentieth-century world that genuinely grappled with the question of how to turn the populism of the nineteenth century into the democracy of the twentieth century through the structuring and standardizing that efficiency provided. Though this kind of efficiency will not be our tool, not least because of the racism intrinsic within it, the serious attempts of its earliest proponents to find a balance—to create a structure rigid enough to produce and disseminate a kind of health that was not utterly subjective while remaining *also* flexible, socially responsible, and egalitarian—might inspire us to do the same.

Notes

INTRODUCTION

1 "Conference on the Standardization of Hospital Practice," March 1, 1915.
2 Baldwin to Gilbreth, March 4, 1916.
3 On the question of what germ theory required and how this was worked out, see Tomes, *The Gospel of Germs*.
4 Nock, "Efficiency and the High-Brow."
5 Gilbreth and Gilbreth, "Hospital Study."
6 See Rosenberg, "The Tyranny of Diagnosis"; Vogel and Rosenberg, *The Therapeutic Revolution*; and Warner, *The Therapeutic Perspective*.
7 Pool and Bancroft were themselves accomplished efficiency experts. In addition to becoming well known in efficiency circles, they also wrote on systematizing surgery. See, e.g., Pool and Bancroft, "Systematization of a Surgical Service."
8 Gilbreth, "Untitled Speech," 18. See also, e.g., "Secretary" to Abraham Flexner, March 9, 1914.
9 Gilbreth, "Untitled Speech," 18–19.
10 Dickinson was a prolific contributor to the medical efficiency literature, even if Gilbreth regarded him as something of a dilettante. See, e.g., Dickinson, "Hospital Efficiency from the Standpoint of the Hospital Surgeon," and "Standardization of Surgery." He is better known now, though, for his work in sexology research and eugenics and for his medical drawings and illustrations and later his sculptures. See, e.g., his work with Lura Beam, *A Thousand Marriages* and *The Single Woman*. The close relationship between eugenics and efficiency is described especially cogently in Currell and Cogdell, *Popular Eugenics*.
11 See, e.g., Flexner, "Adjusting the College to American Life," 363–65.
12 For the pre-efficiency state of affairs, see especially Warner, *The Therapeutic Perspective*, and also Rosenberg, "The Tyranny of Diagnosis."
13 Flexner, *Medical Education*, 5. John Harley Warner has addressed in depth the question of how and why science entered medicine twice over; see Warner, "Science in Medicine," and "The History of Science and the Sciences of Medicine." See also

the important work of Steve Sturdy and Roger Cooter, who make a similar point in "Science, Scientific Management and the Transformation of Medicine in Britain."
14. Richard Lindstrom offers a more nuanced exception to the historiography; see Lindstrom, "'They All Believe.'"
15. See especially Lindstrom's exceptional attempts to recover these voices. Lindstrom, "'They All Believe.'"
16. Tarbell, "Fear of Efficiency, 21.
17. Gilbreth, "Untitled Speech," 18. A more general discussion of scientific management takes place in Rosmary Stevens's *In Sickness and in Wealth*; she implicitly notes (75–79) the desire of surgeons to achieve an autonomy and authority entirely of their own. In this vein, see also Susan Reverby's "Stealing the Golden Eggs," a study of Ernest Codman, who was a Gilbreth devotee. Joel Howell has a much more thorough discussion of Gilbreth's studies but ultimately attributes the significance of efficiency in medicine to Robert Latou Dickinson, a Gilbreth devotee. See Howell, *Technology in the Hospital*.
18. In the details, their views were in fact rather disparate, but the uniting factor, of basic medical ineffectiveness, was a constant. See Illich, *Medical Nemesis*; McKeown, *The Role of Medicine*; Cochrane, *Efficiency and Effectiveness*.
19. See, e.g., Starr, *The Social Transformation of American Medicine*; E. R. Brown, *Rockefeller Medicine Men*; Berliner, *A System of Scientific Medicine*, as well as "New Light on the Flexner Report"; and Markowitz and Rosner, "Doctors in Crisis." Robert Weiss and Lynn Miller also offer a breakdown of these claims in "The Social Transformation of American Medical Education," as does Eliot Freidson in his *Profession of Medicine*. In a 1990 editorial that can only be described as an exasperated outburst, Thomas Bonner criticized these kinds of accounts that read early twentieth-century medicine as fundamentally about power acquisition. He accused them of "presentism," suggesting that they had flattened the nuances of the early twentieth century period in their attempt to describe them in the terms set by the late twentieth century's preoccupation with capitalism, technocracy, and professionalization. See Bonner, "Abraham Flexner and the Historians."
20. Starr, *The Social Transformation of American Medicine*.
21. Braverman, *Labor and Monopoly Capital*. For a useful summary of the historiography, see Chris Wright's "Taylorism Reconsidered."
22. As Roger Cooter summed it up in a 2004 historiographical essay, although we may struggle to put shape to what medicine is, and thus how or what we study when we study it (it is, he quoted John Pickstone, really more of a "convenient omnibus term" encompassing a wide variety of practices, people, and ideas), we can at least say with confidence that "at root medicine is about power: 'the power of doctors and of patients, of institutions such as churches, charities, insurance companies, or pharmaceutical manufacturers, and especially governments, in peacetime or in war.'" Cooter, "'Framing' the End of the Social History of Medicine," 312. Cooter here quotes Pickstone's essay "Medicine, Society and the State."
23. See especially Reverby, "Stealing the Golden Eggs," and Crenner, "Organizational Reform and Professional Dissent." References to the failures of efficiency are a common theme in history of medicine texts. Classic among these are Stevens, *In Sickness*

and in Wealth, and Starr, *The Social Transformation of American Medicine*. But there are also useful corrections to this view, which do not call themselves efficiency but are in every way consistent with, or predecessors to, efficiency efforts. See, in this vein, e.g., Warner, *The Therapeutic Perspective*, and Rosenberg, "The Tyranny of Diagnosis."

24 Sociological work on standardization has been quite useful, although it does not, by and large, consider efficiency to any great degree. See, e.g., Timmermans and Berg, *The Gold Standard*. On the implications of scientific management in British medicine over a similar period, see Sturdy and Cooter, "Science, Scientific Management and the Transformation of Medicine in Britain." For an examination of the unexpectedly intertwining mores, practices, materials, and approaches of industry, efficiency, and medicine in European countries, see Schlich, *Surgery, Science and Industry* and his case study "Trauma Surgery and Traffic Policy in Germany."

25 The classic articulation that Taylorism amounted to little in practice is probably the work of Daniel Nelson, *Frederick W. Taylor and the Rise of Scientific Management*. See also Wright, "Taylorism Reconsidered."

26 See Nelson, Frederick W. Taylor and the Rise of Scientific Management; see also, e.g., Kraines, "Brandeis' Philosophy of Scientific Management."

27 Haber, *Efficiency and Uplift*. See also Aitken, *Scientific Management in Action*; Kanigel, *The One Best Way*; Hounshell, *From the American System to Mass Production*; Alexander, *The Mantra of Efficiency*; and Rabinbach, *The Human Motor*.

28 Hays, *Conservation and the Gospel of Efficiency*.

29 Dewey, or Dui—first name, Melvil—as he chose for a time to be more efficiently known, was not successful in this venture. Rather than reify his position as an efficiency figure, this phonetic fix flopped, cementing the retrospective view that the eccentric in this case had not been the English language but Dui himself. For more on Dewey, see, e.g., Wiegand, "Dewey Declassified," and Fields and Connell, "Classification and the Definition of a Discipline."

30 See, e.g., Graham, "Domesticating Efficiency."

31 "Movies to Help Baseball Players Economize Force."

32 Edward Earle Purinton was first brought to the attention of readers of the *Independent* in October 1914. The editors, in their "Just a Word" column, announced that the magazine's November 30 issue would be an "efficiency number" and would highlight Purinton's work, since his "writing on this . . . topic has attracted the attention of millions of people." On December 21 of that same year, Purinton inaugurated the *Independent*'s "Efficiency Question Box" column (later renamed "Mr. Purinton's Efficiency Question Box" as his fame grew), which invited readers to send in questions on the "subject of personal efficiency as it relates to health, work and business." In the first edition alone, questions ran an illustrative gambit, from practical inquiries about instituting greater efficiency in the use of delivery wagons, to a plead for help in curing "two years of nervous breakdown," to the efficiency method by which a man might find his "supreme talent." See also Purinton, *Efficient Living* and *Personal Efficiency in Business*. For more background on Purinton, see Alexander, *The Mantra of Efficiency*.

33 See, e.g., Durkin, "The (Re)production Craze," and Lichtenstein, "Domestic Novels of the 1920s."

34 The examples describing efficiency as autocratic are many. See, e.g., Lalvani, *Photography, Vision, and the Production of Modern Bodies*; Corwin, "Picturing Efficiency"; Tenner, "The Technological Imperative"; Mandell, *Making Good Time*; Montgomery, *Workers' Control in America*; Cohen, *Making a New Deal*; Nadworny, *Scientific Management and the Unions*; Aitken, *Scientific Management in Action*.

35 As Rosemary Stevens put it in her formidable 1989 study of American hospitals, "From the medical point of view the standardization movement was . . . both aristocratic (elitist) and democratic (or all-inclusive). . . . From its beginnings to the present, hospital accreditation has embodied mixed messages" (Stevens, *In Sickness and in Wealth*, 52).

36 Lindstrom, "'They All Believe,'" and Gainty, "'Going after the High-Brows.'"

37 Nock, "Efficiency and the High-Brow."

38 Link, *Forging Global Fordism*. Even Taylor has occasionally seen glimpses of rehabilitation. See, e.g., Nyland, "Taylorism, John R. Commons, and the Hoxie Report." Perhaps best known are Daniel Nelson's works on Taylor; see Nelson, *Frederick W. Taylor and the Rise of Scientific Management*, and "Scientific Management and the Workplace." See also Nyland, *Reduced Worktime and the Management of Production*; Schachter, "Democracy, Scientific Management and Urban Reform."

39 Barton, "Concerning Calvin Coolidge," 8.

40 A good starting point for discussion of the standardization considerations of the National Medical Association is Gamble, "The Negro Hospital Renaissance."

41 Green, "Annual Address of the President," 215–16.

42 Tomes, "Comment," 374. She credits this phrase to Steven Mihm and quotes it from Beckert et al., "Interchange: The History of Capitalism," 515.

1. THE PRODUCT

1 Codman, "The Product of a Hospital," 491.
2 Gilbreth, "Hospital Efficiency."
3 Starr, *The Social Transformation of American Medicine*.
4 Starr, *The Social Transformation of American Medicine*, 22.
5 For a fuller discussion of Codman, see Reverby, "Stealing the Golden Eggs," and Crenner, "Organizational Reform and Professional Dissent." Codman's search for a product led to his founding the "End Result Hospital" in Boston's Beacon Hill, which he ran between 1911 and 1917. Setting surgical outcomes as the product by which he and his colleagues might be measured, Codman recorded his hospital's "end results" in detail, subdividing surgical errors and distinguishing those caused by a failed product from those caused by disease itself. The success of this pursuit, though, has remained uncertain. For example, S. S. Goldwater wrote to Codman in 1913 to voice concern over a particular follow-up aspect of the end-result system employed at his own New York Hospital, noting that "efficiency tests . . . are always of some value [but] sometimes it is necessary to put the measuring rod on the testing method itself." For more on the specifics of Codman's emphasis on product, see Codman, *A Study in Hospital Efficiency*. See also Gainty, "The Autobiographical *Shoulder* of Ernest Amory Codman"; Berwick, "E. A. Codman and the Rhetoric of Battle."

6 This vision of efficiency became popular among critics during the 1930s, especially embedded in criticisms that blamed the severe economic downtown of the Great Depression on the overproduction that was mass production—and thus also efficiency's—legacy. See, e.g., Foster, "Planning in a Free Country"; Filene, "The Minimum Wage and Efficiency"; Brookings, *The Way Forward*; Leven, Moulton, and Warburton, *America's Capacity to Consume*; Foster and Catchings, *Business without a Buyer*; and Tugwell, *Industry's Coming of Age*. Later studies picked up this criticism as well, especially the Marxist labor histories of the 1970s. See especially Braverman, *Labor and Monopoly Capital*.

7 The Gilbreths described "happiness minutes" in the context of their studies of fatigue. "The aim of life is happiness," they wrote, "no matter how we differ as to what true happiness means. Fatigue elimination, starting as it does from a desire to conserve human life and to eliminate enormous waste, must increase 'Happiness Minutes,' no matter what else it does, or it has failed in its fundamental aim." See Gilbreth and Gilbreth, *Fatigue Study*, 149–50. It is easy to read this, and many have, as one of the Gilbreths' more nefarious strategies to acquire the kind of buy-in from workers that would make them more amenable to being rationalized in the first place. For this interpretation and an explanation of Lillian Gilbreth's use of the term "happiness minutes," see Graham, "Domesticating Efficiency." Similar discussions arise in Noble, *America by Design*, and E. Brown, *The Corporate Eye*.

8 Ford describes this manufacturing system in his autobiography. See Ford and Crowther, "My Life and Work: Chapter IV." See also Shumard, "Correspondence."

9 In his introduction to the second edition of *Principles of Scientific Management*, Frederick Winslow Taylor notes that he will convince the reader that "management is a true science, resting upon clearly defined laws, rules and principles as a foundation." Taylor, *Principles of Scientific Management*, 7.

10 This paradigmatic tension is made clear in the efficiency literature. See D. Nelson, *Frederick W. Taylor and the Rise of Scientific Management*, and "Scientific Management and the Workplace." See also E. Brown, *The Corporate Eye*; Lindstrom, "'They All Believe'"; Curtis, "Images of Efficiency"; Alexander, *The Mantra of Efficiency*; Noble, *America by Design*.

11 Rabinbach, *The Human Motor*. See also Hyde, *Bodies of Law*, 34–47.

12 See Vogel and Rosenberg, *The Therapeutic Revolution*, and Warner, *The Therapeutic Perspective*.

13 Hyde, *Bodies of Law*, 34.

14 See, e.g., Derickson, "Physiological Science and Scientific Management in the Progressive Era."

15 Kellogg, *The Stomach*, 3. See also Bauch, "The Extensible Digestive System."

16 Bauch, *A Geography of Digestion*.

17 See Kellogg, *The Itinerary of a Breakfast*, 88–90.

18 Fletcher, *Fletcherism*. For discussions of waste in the context of efficiency, see, e.g., Alexander, *The Mantra of Efficiency*. Exemplary of articulations of efficiency at the time is the Robert Hoxie's report on scientific management: "Scientific management is a system devised by industrial engineers for the purpose of subserving the common interests of employers, workmen and society at large through the elimination

of avoidable wastes, the general improvement of the processes and methods of production, and the just and scientific distribution of the product." Hoxie, "Why Organized Labor Opposes Scientific Management," 482–83.
19 Kellogg did not by any means qualify as a conventional medical figure. Indeed, Abraham Flexner's 1910 evaluation of medical education excoriated the "san" for its influence over its affiliate, the American Medical Missionary School. Flexner bitingly noted that medical students at the AMMS operated "under the limitations of the theories approved by the Sanitarium authorities," which "hardly cultivates... a critical and investigative spirit." To this, Rowland Harris, the secretary of the faculty, replied rather hotly, "I do not quite understand what is meant by your statement. I do not think any different opinions are held by the physicians of this College in regard to etiology, pathology and symptomatology of disease than are held by physicians all over the world" (R. H. Harris to Flexner, April 24, 1910).
20 Kellogg, *The Itinerary of a Breakfast*, 73.
21 Kellogg, *The Itinerary of a Breakfast*, 9.
22 Kellogg, *The Itinerary of a Breakfast*, 9.
23 For a complete discussion of germ theory, see Tomes, *The Gospel of Germs*, and Leavitt, *Typhoid Mary*. Concern about bacteria was not peculiar to digestion. It registered a national fear of microbiotic enemies. Indeed, in the early twentieth century, the belief that any bacteria was bad bacteria was manifested in the contemporary design of "modern" hospitals, where architects were tasked with designing out of existence the bacterium's preferred hiding places. Fears of bacteria also gave rise to changed designs of bathrooms and kitchens—those places perceived as dirtiest in the domestic sphere. And in the world of consumer goods, fear of bacteria paired nicely with trending industrial design, producing everyday household objects with smooth, shiny, and easily cleaned surfaces. The *streamline moderne* movement, which produced buildings that looked like boats, cars modeled on airplanes, and in at least one famous case, a pencil sharpener that looked like it could fly, owes as much to early twentieth-century fears about bacteria as it does the physics of flight. See, e.g., Lupton and Miller, *The Bathroom, the Kitchen and the Aesthetics of Waste*, and Cogdell, *Eugenic Design*.
24 Kellogg, *Itinerary of a Breakfast*, 65.
25 Boston Women's Health Book Collective, *Our Bodies, Ourselves*. See also, e.g., Dye, "History of Childbirth in America."
26 Duden, *The Woman Beneath the Skin*, 28–29. On childbirth's "industrialization," see also Haire, "The Cultural Warping of Childbirth"; Plante, "Mommy, What Did You Do in the Industrial Revolution?"; J. C. Jones, "Idealized and Industrialized Labor."
27 On medicalization, the classic accounts are probably Starr, *The Social Transformation of American Medicine*; Freidson, *Profession of Medicine*; and E. R. Brown, *Rockefeller Medicine Men*. In thoughtful response to these classic works, see, e.g., Rose, "Beyond Medicalisation," and Williams and Calnan, "The 'Limits' of Medicalization?" For examples of the complications of the medicalization of childbirth, see Leavitt, *Brought to Bed*, and Tone, *Devices and Desires*. For a good discussion of medicalization and its work in reproduction, see Tone, "Medicalizing Reproduction"; Olszynko-Gryn, *A Woman's Right to Know*; Morgen, *Into Our Own Hands*; Kline, *Bodies of Knowledge*; Murphy, *Seizing the Means of Reproduction*; J. Nelson, *More than Medicine*.

28 This is well known. See especially Judith Walzer Leavitt's discussion in *Brought to Bed*.
29 Caton, "Who Said Childbirth Is Natural?" See also Paula Michaels's excellent study in which she writes, "Dick-Read believed that as a natural, normal physiological function, akin to the expulsive capabilities of the bowels, childbirth could not have been designed in such a way as to be an inherently painful process" (Michaels, *Lamaze*, 19).
30 See Dick-Read, *Natural Childbirth*. Unlike obstetrician Joseph DeLee, Dick-Read is celebrated as a key figure in the natural childbirth movement. Primitive birth indeed comes up quite a lot in the literature, sometimes celebrated, sometimes denigrated; see, e.g., "Hints for Hospital Superintendents."
31 Dick-Read, *Natural Childbirth*, 86.
32 Richardson, "'Better Babies.'"
33 DeLee "The Prophylactic Forceps Operation," 41.
34 DeLee "The Prophylactic Forceps Operation," 41.
35 DeLee, "The Chicago Lying-in Hospital and Dispensary," 386.
36 DeLee "The Prophylactic Forceps Operation." See also Gainty, "A Bit of Hollywood in the Operating Room" and "'Items for Criticism.'"
37 Gainty, "A Bit of Hollywood in the Operating Room."
38 This is a well-known phenomenon, quite usefully summed up in Michaels, *Lamaze*, as well as in Cogdell, *Eugenic Design* and in Moscucci, "Holistic Obstetrics." Dick-Read himself sets the "eugenic minimum" at four children in *Motherhood in the Post-War World*. For background, see Leavitt, "Science Enters the Birthing Room," and Leavitt, "Joseph B. DeLee and the Practice of Preventive Obstetrics."
39 DeLee, "Before the Baby Comes," 35.
40 For a full discussion of the Chicago Maternity Center and the work DeLee did among the urban poor in Chicago, see Kline, "Back to Bed"; Gainty, "'Items for Criticism'"; Kline, "How to Train an Obstetrician."
41 McEvoy, "Our Streamlined Baby," 15–16.
42 See Williams, "A Criticism of Certain Tendencies in American Obstetrics," and "Medical Education and the Midwife Problem in the United States," 1. Williams's views get a full and useful airing in Leavitt, *Brought to Bed*.
43 See Gainty, "'Items for Criticism'"; Ostherr, *Medical Visions*; and the edited volume by Orgeron, Orgeron, and Streible, *Learning with the Lights Off*.
44 DeLee, "The Prophylactic Forceps Operation," 41.
45 DeLee, *The Science and Art of Obstetrics*.
46 Liebes to Joseph, April 28, 1963.
47 DeLee, "The Motion Picture in Obstetric Teaching," and DeLee, "Sound Motion Pictures in Obstetrics."
48 M. Davis, "Dispensary and Outpatient Work," 293.
49 "Moving Sidewalks and Other Luxuries," 273.
50 There is a great deal of discussion in the scholarly literature on this phenomenon. The classics are surely Starr, *Social Transformation of American Medicine*; Stevens, *In Sickness and in Wealth*; Rosenberg, *The Care of Strangers*; Howell, *Technology in the Hospital*; Vogel, *The Invention of the Modern Hospital*. See also Kisacky, *Rise of the Modern Hospital*. An interesting additional contribution is Getzen, "A 'Brand Name Firm' Theory of Medical Group Practice."

51 Hirshberg, "Cities Should Maintain Free Diagnostic Clinics."
52 Chenery, "Ford Hospital Upsets the Old Medical Traditions." See also Cabot, "Better Doctoring for Less Money."
53 Hornsby, "How a Great Clinic Works," 335.
54 Cabot, "Better Doctoring for Less Money," 81. See also M. Davis, "Group Medicine."
55 Mayo, "Nature, Value and Necessity of Teamwork in a Hospital," 2.
56 For a fuller breakdown on the hospital architecture of this period, see the excellent discussion in Kisacky, *Rise of the Modern Hospital*. See also A. Adams, *Medicine by Design*.
57 Plummer later designed a separate energy plant for the clinic, to support his next building project, which is still extant and is known now as the Plummer Building. See "Plummer Building," 17.
58 Richard Beard's effusive review of the new building describes its ingenious additions floor by floor. See Beard, "The Mayo Clinic Building, Rochester, Minnesota."
59 "Formal Opening of Clinic Attracts Hundreds of People."
60 "Formal Opening of Clinic Attracts Hundreds of People."
61 "The Mayo Clinic Building Is Formally Opened."
62 Cabot, "Better Doctoring for Less Money," 43.

2. THE FACTORY

1 Link, *Forging Global Fordism*.
2 Link, *Forging Global Fordism*, 39. See also Esch, *The Color Line and the Assembly Line*, 1–3.
3 Antonio and Bonnano, "A New Global Capitalism?" See also Gramsci, "From 'Americanism and Fordism.'"
4 Antonio and Bonnano, "A New Global Capitalism?," 35. The classic of this genre is probably Braverman, *Labor and Monopoly Capital*.
5 As William Greenleaf insisted in his book lauding the philanthropic work of Ford and his children, Ford really *was* "actuated by a philanthropic impulse." It was just that his upbringing in the "rural and self-sufficient America" of the late nineteenth century made him hide this impulse, masking its manifestations in a set of "personal predilections and crotchets." See Greenleaf, *From These Beginnings*, 1.
6 See, e.g., Kisacky, *Rise of the Modern Hospital*, 235–95.
7 Crowther, "The Real Story of Ford's Hospital," 540.
8 See Kisacky, *Rise of the Modern Hospital*, 235–95; see also Howell, *Technology in the Hospital*, which is a classic. References to the uptick in technologizing hospitals can also be found in, e.g., Stevens, *In Sickness and in Wealth*; Starr, *The Social Transformation of American Medicine*.
9 Link, *Forging Global Fordism*, 7.
10 Kisacky, *Rise of the Modern Hospital*, 293.
11 Chimes, "The History of the Henry Ford Hospital," 30. This story is described also in Painter, *Henry Ford Hospital*, 29.
12 This story is well described throughout the literature, but see, e.g., Meyer, "Adapting the Immigrant to the Line."
13 Greenleaf, *From These Beginnings*, 39. It is difficult to discover which article this may be: the most antagonistic article in the *Detroit Times* suggested only that the "failure of

[the] merger" with the Harper Hospital had given impetus to a scheme for the city to be turned over to the city of Detroit. See, e.g., "Mayor Plans to Have City Take Over and Operate Detroit General Hospital." A common suggestion in newspapers during May 1914 was that Ford would take over the project in order to avoid this merger going through. See, e.g., "Officials Believe Hospital's Offer Will Be Accepted."

14 This story is repeated throughout the literature. See, e.g., Gilbert, "A Woman Interviews Henry Ford."
15 Greenleaf, *From These Beginnings*, 32. Ford repeatedly describes his intent to turn his hospital over from "cure" to "prevention." See "Curing and Preventing" in Ford and Crowther, *Today and Tomorrow*, 186–92.
16 McFeeley, "Will Spend Millions in New Hospital," 1.
17 Reminiscences of Dr. F. Janney Smith, 17.
18 On eating grass, see Reminiscences of William J. Cameron, described also in Greenleaf, *From These Beginnings*, 195. Ford and Crowther, "Greatest Goal in Disease Prevention, Asserts Ford." Indeed, a later iteration of this prevention theme, in which Ford described his as-yet unfinished hospital as being focused explicitly on the prevention of cancer (probably also through diet, though Ford did not publicly specify), also never came to pass. On Ford's intentions with reference to cancer, see McFeeley, "Will Spend Millions," 1; see also "Who Names the Ford Hospital Wins Big Honors," 36.
19 McFeeley, "Will Spend Millions," 1.
20 McFeeley, "Will Spend Millions," 1.
21 Hooker, "Ford's Sociology Department."
22 Hooker, "Ford's Sociology Department," 49.
23 See Bates, *The Making of Black Detroit*, and Esch, *The Color Line and the Assembly Line*, for a fuller picture of Ford's egalitarian-eugenicist attitude toward Black workers.
24 This assessment is offered in L. Adams, "Review: Beth Tompkins Bates, *The Making of Black Detroit in the Age of Henry Ford*," 616.
25 McFeeley, "Ford Consumptives Cured at Work," 1.
26 Cobley, *Modernism and the Culture of Efficiency*, 38–76. See also Pietrykowski, "Fordism at Ford."
27 Babson, "What Henry Ford Really Said to Roger Babson," 61.
28 Babson, "What Henry Ford Really Said to Roger Babson," 61.
29 Link, *Forging Global Fordism*, 39–40.
30 "Gospel of Cleanliness and Thrift," 5.
31 Lee, "The So-Called Profit Sharing System."
32 Lee, "The So-Called Profit Sharing System."
33 Newspapers were replete with stories about how the Ford investigators did not judge but assisted these workers and their families to improve their lot, reach their potential, *and* therefore get their share of the Ford profits. Families down on their luck who ended up in a shared and dirty rooming house—one couple with a new baby had just a kitchen to call their home—were driven around to find more suitable accommodations. And then there were the "two Slav boys" who had been denied the $5 day wage because of their living conditions: a room with four beds used by its fourteen occupants in shifts. The investigator drove them to a "pigsty at

the edge of town": a non-subtle demonstration of what he thought of their rooming arrangement. That apparently turned them around. "The lesson had been learned. They are getting the increase," the article trumpeted, concluding that "Ford workers are . . . not being driven—just shown the way and that is the way they take [it], 99 per cent of the time. . . . Once they know and live the standard set for them they will never again go back to the olden days of slavery to insanitation." See "Gospel of Cleanliness and Thrift," 5.

34 For contemporary accounts, see, e.g., "Henry Ford's Latest Action," 6, and its follow-up, "Ford Profit-Sharing Plan Is Explained," 2. For particularly useful readings of the $5 day wage in historical retrospect and its place in Fordism, see Meyer, "Adapting the Immigrant to the Line." Foote, Whatley, and Wright, "Arbitraging a Discriminatory Labor Market," is especially useful for articulating how Ford's commitment to equal wages played out as part of longer, larger discriminatory logics. As labor unions acquired more power and Ford's strategies came to seem increasingly coercive, worker unrest and strikes became more frequent. These upheavals culminated in the Hunger Strike at Ford's River Rouge Plant in 1931 and, eventually in the 1940s, unionization. See Cobley, *Modernism and the Culture of Efficiency*, 38–76.

35 For more on the conflicted nature of Ford's sociological department and its policies, see, e.g., Loizides and Sonnad, "Fordist Applied Research in the Era of the Five-Dollar Day."

36 Ford and Crowther, *Today and Tomorrow*, 186–87. As described by some architectural historians, some of these elements were the result of the experience with the war wounded. Hospitals that resembled factories, at least insofar as patients traversed through as if on an assembly line, became well known as a solution to the problem of managing the large numbers of wounded soldiers, nearly all of them in need of urgent attention, who arrived at the field hospitals. Though wartime came with many lessons, World War I did not, of course, invent medical efficiency.

37 M. Davis, "Dispensary and Outpatient Work." See also, e.g., Kisacky, *Rise of the Modern Hospital*, 235–95; Howell, *Technology in the Hospital*; Gainty, "Why Wait?"

38 Crowther, "The Real Story of Ford's Hospital," 543.

39 Du Puy, "Henry Ford, of Dearborn," 10.

40 "Ford Hospital Aims to Put Health Service on Economic Business Basis." See also Ford and Crowther, *Today and Tomorrow*, 186–92. As Stefan Link points out, this more populist vision of how mass production came to be is often buried in analyses that depict Fordism as a top-down rather than bottom-up affair. Link, *Forging Global Fordism*, 19–50.

41 Chenery, "Ford Hospital Upsets the Old Medical Traditions."

42 Ahuja, "Fordism in the Hospital," 419. The hospital as factory motif is well described in Kisacky, *Rise of the Modern Hospital*, 235–95.

43 In practical part, this reflected the fact that private rooms contained disease within their four walls, as opposed to the ward system, where patients with the same diseases or illnesses would be housed together. A full ward meant that a new patient with that same illness would be turned away. Likewise, it meant that wards that were not full had unused, and unusable, beds. Private rooms thus were preferred. For a full description, see Kisacky, *Rise of the Modern Hospital*, 277–79.

44 Wright, "Dimensions of Private Rooms."
45 See Gilbreth and Gilbreth, "Hospital Study."
46 See, e.g., the discussions of standardizing hospital objects and architecture in the "Home-Made Hospital Appliances" column in *Modern Hospital*, which ran over multiple issues in 1914 (which is discussed in greater detail in chapter 3).
47 Painter, *Henry Ford Hospital*, 28.
48 "Ford Hospital Aims to Put Health Service on Economic Business Basis." See also Chenery, "Ford Hospital Upsets the Old Medical Traditions."
49 For more on the rise of group practice, see especially Stevens, *In Sickness and in Wealth*, 17–51.
50 M. Davis, "Dispensary and Outpatient Work," 293.
51 Ahuja, "Fordism in the Hospital," 417.
52 Chenery, "Ford Hospital Upsets the Old Medical Traditions."
53 "Objects to Ethics of Ford's Hospital," 12.
54 "Surgeons Attack Ford Hospital System," 1.
55 "Business Man's Businesslike Hospital," 16.
56 "Ford Hospital Head Quits Surgeons' Body," 1.
57 Cabot, "Better Doctoring for Less Money," 76–78, 81.
58 Cabot, "Better Doctoring for Less Money," 78.
59 This method is described in an article in the *American Magazine* about how a young surgeon had secured "a professional income [of] more than twenty thousand dollars" by building up his wealthy clientele, through word-of-mouth, so that he could build up a good living more quickly. Though the story is eye-opening on the subjects of medical fee-setting and surgical practice, it is obviously meant to be inspirational—a paragon of successful business practices. See Woolley, "A Successful Surgeon's Own Story," 80–82.
60 Crowther, "The Real Story of Ford's Hospital," 543–44.
61 Ford and Crowther, "Greatest Goal in Disease Prevention." See also "Ford Hospital in Detroit."
62 There is a small bit of uncertainty here, since in 1925, the Michigan State Medical Society ran an article suggesting that Ford had changed this fixed pricing so that there were maximum spending limits but no longer specific prices. Newspaper articles, however, continued to run this piece, suggesting that the fixed pricing format was still in effect as late as 1926. See Ford and Crowther, "Greatest Goal in Disease Prevention," for example.
63 Crowther, "The Real Story of Ford's Hospital." See also Greenleaf, *From These Beginnings*, 45–46. In 1928, this plan was mimicked at a Los Angeles hospital. See "Hospital Cost Standardized," A8.
64 Chenery, "Ford Hospital Upsets the Old Medical Traditions."
65 Cabot, "Better Doctoring for Less Money," 43. William Mayo stated that the Mayo Clinic never turned patients away and did about 30 percent of its work for charity. See "Work of Drs. Mayo Now Perpetuated for People's Good," 8.
66 Chenery, "Ford Hospital Upsets the Old Medical Traditions." Ford himself had been aghast when his wife Clara Ford was charged $1,300 for an operation.
67 "Surgeons Attack Ford Hospital System."

68 Chenery, "Ford Hospital Upsets the Old Medical Traditions."
69 Du Puy, "Henry Ford, of Dearborn," 10.
70 Link, *Forging Global Fordism*, 27–28.
71 Link, *Forging Global Fordism*, 36–37.
72 Shumard, "Correspondence: Foresight of Henry Ford."
73 Cobley, *Modernism and the Culture of Efficiency*, 38–76.
74 Shumard, "Correspondence: Foresight of Henry Ford."
75 Cobley, *Modernism and the Culture of Efficiency*, 38–76.
76 Ford and Crowther, "My Life and Work: Chapter IV," 35.
77 Chenery, "Ford Hospital Upsets the Old Medical Traditions."
78 Link, *Forging Global Fordism*, 28–29. Link convincingly argues that Ford's success is in part related to the distinctively populist politics of the Midwest, which in turn was a result of its peculiar history of industrialization.
79 "A Business Man's Businesslike Hospital."
80 Du Puy, "Henry Ford, of Dearborn."
81 "Retail Prices: 1913 to December 1920," *Bulletin of the United States Bureau of Labor Statistics*, Washington, DC: Government Printing Office, 1922, 161–63.
82 Painter, *Henry Ford Hospital*, 51. This working method caught on, with the hospital literature generally assenting that "adequate salaries and good living conditions were a wise expenditure," though less, as one article opined, because of the stabilizing effects on the hospital workforce and more for the more ephemeral "*esprit de corps*" they tended to inculcate. See, e.g., R. G. Broderick, "The Effect of the Eight Hour Day on the Hospital Budget."
83 See, e.g., Cooper, "The Henry Ford Hospital in Time of War," and Martin, "Henry Ford Hospital in Time of Peace."
84 Greenleaf, *From These Beginnings*, 68–69.
85 Greenleaf, *From These Beginnings*, 69.
86 "Hospitals Big Asset to City."
87 V. Thomas, *Partners of the Heart*, 38.
88 Niebuhr, *The Negro in Detroit, Section 6: Health*, 13. Jeffrey Rodengen's history of the Ford Hospital describes, on the other hand, the experiences of one of the first Black employees at the Ford Hospital, Wilma Gandy, who joined the staff as a ward clerk in 1955. Rodengen, *Henry Ford Health System*, 95.
89 Niebuhr, *The Negro in Detroit, Section 6: Health*, 13–17.
90 See the discussion on Black patients in Rodengen, *Henry Ford Health System*, 104–6
91 Esch, *The Color Line and the Assembly Line*, 84–86.
92 Bates, *The Making of Black Detroit*, 69–91.
93 The newspapers covered the trial extensively, in part because Clarence Darrow had arrived in town to defend Sweet and his codefendants. See, e.g., "Ten Are Held for Murder in Race Conflict," and "Darrow Will Defend Sweet." See also Bates, *The Making of Black Detroit*, 93.
94 Bates, *The Making of Black Detroit*, 2.
95 The phrase is well known. Here I draw especially on Esch, *The Color Line and the Assembly Line*, 1.
96 For a fuller discussion, see E. R. Brown, *Rockefeller Medicine Men*.

3. THE STANDARD

1. "Home-Made Hospital Appliances," July 1914, 52.
2. "Home-Made Hospital Appliances," November 1914, 337.
3. Washburn, "Standardized Home-Made Appliances," 133.
4. "Home-Made Hospital Appliances," July 1914, 51.
5. "Home-Made Hospital Appliances," October 1914, 267.
6. "Home-Made Hospital Appliances," October 1914, 267.
7. "Home-Made Hospital Appliances," July 1914, 42.
8. "Conference on the Standardization of Hospital Practice," 10.
9. "Conference on the Standardization of Hospital Practice," 3–4.
10. A point beautifully made by Ruth Schwartz Cowan in her classic *More Work for Mother*.
11. This was one of the arguments that Codman made in *A Study in Hospital Efficiency*, 133–34.
12. For a discussion of other organizations also attempting to elevate surgical standards, see "Editorial: The College of Surgeons." See also Board of Regents Meeting Minutes, May 15, 1913; L. Davis, *Fellowship of Surgeons*; Young, "On the Economics of New Medical Titles," 660; and "Graft at the Bottom."
13. See, e.g., the "Joint Commission History Timeline."
14. For general discussions of defining standards, see Bowker and Star, *Sorting Things Out*; Timmermans and Epstein, "A World of Standards"; and Lampland and Star, *Standards and Their Stories*, 3–34.
15. Bowker and Star, *Sorting Things Out*, 1–18.
16. The classic source is Braverman, *Labor and Monopoly Capital*.
17. See, e.g., the explanation in Beaudreau and Taylor, "Why Did the Roosevelt Administration."
18. See Tarbell, *The History of the Standard Oil Company*.
19. Timmermans and Epstein, "A World of Standards"; White, *The Republic for Which It Stands*; Adelstein, "'Islands of Conscious Power'"; Lamoreaux, "The Problem of Bigness." See also Chandler, *The Visible Hand*; Granitz and Klein, "Monopolization by 'Raising Rivals' Costs.'"
20. Though still not fully hashed out even in the early twentieth century, this was a view that was distinctively tied to the nineteenth century. See, e.g., Rosenberg, "The Tyranny of Diagnosis."
21. Flexner, *Medical Education*, 3.
22. "A Physician: The Plight of the Family Doctor," 7.
23. See Codman, *A Study in Hospital Efficiency*, 1, for a description of his hospital. See also Gainty, "The Autobiographical *Shoulder* of Ernest Amory Codman."
24. Nock, "Efficiency and the High-Brow." See also Gilbreth, "Motion Study in Surgery," 25–27; and for background, see Gainty, "Going after the High-Brows."
25. "Appendectomy."
26. "Home-Made Hospital Appliances," July 1914, 51–52.
27. Valentine, "Application of Principles of Organization to Hospital Service," 262.
28. Taylor, *The Principles of Scientific Management*.

29 "Conference on the Standardization of Hospital Practice," 12.
30 See especially Flexner, *The American College: A Criticism*.
31 See, e.g., Flexner, "Aristocratic and Democratic Education"; Flexner, "The German Side of Medical Education"; and Flexner, *The American College*. See also M. R. Harris, *Five Counterrevolutionaries in Higher Education*.
32 See Flexner, "Aristocratic and Democratic Education" and especially "The German Side of Medical Education."
33 Louis Brandeis describes the purchase of Andrew Carnegie's US Steel, in the formation of the Steel Trust, as an example of the desire of monopolies to preserve *inefficiency* in the market, because US Steel had been so efficient that no company could come near its prices. "Because his competitors were unable to rise to his remarkable efficiency, his business career was killed; and the American people were deprived of his ability—his genius—to produce steel cheaply" (Brandeis, "Trusts, Efficiency, and the New Party," 14). For useful background on Brandeis and efficiency, see especially Aldrich, "On the Track of Efficiency."
34 The same was famously true at the Ford Motor Company. Here, too, increasing standardization passed along to consumers a low and, for a decade at least, ever-decreasing price. In each case, efficiency's success in the factory was made manifest in the form of the more egalitarian distribution that lower prices made possible. See Shumard, "Correspondence."
35 See, e.g., Noble, *America by Design*, and Noble, *Forces of Production*. See also Beniger, *The Control Revolution*.
36 Young, "On the Economics of New Medical Titles," 660.
37 Young, "On the Economics of New Medical Titles."
38 Board of Regents Meeting Minutes, May 15, 1913.
39 As pejoratively described in P. M. Jones, "Congress of Surgeons."
40 This is part of the argument, indeed, that suggests that the imposition of standards were, after all, primarily aimed at the hallmarks of professionalization: autonomy and authority. See, e.g., Freidson, *Profession of Medicine* and Starr, *The Social Transformation of American Medicine*.
41 Finney, "The Standardization of the Surgeon," 1437.
42 "Editorial: The College of Surgeons," 91. The Flexner Report is the subject of chapter 4.
43 Brickner, "The College of Surgeons," 234.
44 See, e.g., Brickner, "The College of Surgeons," and "Editorial: The College of Surgeons" that appeared in the *New York Medical Journal*. Compounding this was the complaint, articulated best by the surgeon Ernest Amory Codman, that a number of surgery's leading lights in this period, some of whom were founders of the ACS, had acquired their positions by virtue of their family status and wealth or their prior connections within the medical community or, frequently—as these were often coincident—both. Codman, *The Shoulder*, xx–xxix.
45 Nock, "Efficiency and the High-Brow."
46 Grimm, "Notebooks," reel 32/1.
47 Of this total, 1,999 were white surgeons and one was Daniel Hale Williams, the cofounder of the Black medical organization, the National Medical Association (NMA). For more on Williams, see Gamble, *Making a Place for Ourselves*, 3–34.

48 "1,000 Surgeons to Get Fellowships," *The Montgomery Advertiser*, November 13, 1913, 10.
49 Board of Regents Meeting Minutes, May 15, 1913.
50 "Program of Activity," 11–12.
51 As described in Brickner, "The College of Surgeons." See also Young, "On the Economics of New Medical Titles."
52 As described in Brickner, "The College of Surgeons."
53 These sentiments were common: see Loyal Davis's report of a Philadelphia meeting, in which John Gibbon objected that the College "would establish a class distinction in the United States in imitation of European methods which were distinctly undemocratic" (Davis, *Fellowship of Surgeons*, 75). See also "Editorial: The College of Surgeons"; Brickner, "The College of Surgeons"; Young, "On the Economics of New Medical Titles"; and "Graft at the Bottom."
54 Young, "On the Economics of New Medical Titles," 660.
55 Young, "On the Economics of New Medical Titles," 660. This line of questioning about the nature of organizations like the American College of Surgeons was actually long-standing. At the close of the nineteenth century, when increasing numbers of medical organizations began to form, critics saw in these formations the same sort of pejorative parallel with European aristocracies and their more general desire to "assume superiority . . . over [their] fellows, and therefore to assert exclusiveness in association, rank or privilege." The American antidote to aristocracy, at least according to these commentators, had been found in democracy, which, in medical terms, was here interpreted as a specific guarantee that membership in professional societies was accommodating, not exclusive. That the doors to these societies had been closed to average practitioners, however, and that the medical profession had its own sort of aristocracy was well known ("Exclusiveism and Specialism in Medical Organizations," 14).
56 P. M. Jones, "The American Royal College of Surgeons—J. B. M." See also Jones, "The American Royal Surgical Emporium."
57 P. M. Jones, "The Costume of the College."
58 P. M. Jones, "The Costume of the College."
59 One of the most sacred of prohibitions on the otherwise scanty list of conventional medicine's ethical do's and don'ts in this period was self-promotion. In 1847, the American Medical Association had issued the final word on the subject, with a short booklet outlining the profession's code of ethics. Article I subsection 3 reads: "It is derogatory to the dignity of the profession to resort to public advertisements, or private cards, or handbills, inviting the attention of individuals affected with particular diseases—publicly offering advice and medicine or to publish cases and operations in the daily prints, or suffer such publication to be made; to invite laymen to be present at operations, to boast of cures and remedies, to adduce certificates of skill and success, or to perform any other similar acts. These are the ordinary practices of empirics, and are highly reprehensible in a regular physician" (*Code of Ethics of the American Medical Association Adopted 1847*, 11).
60 P. M. Jones, "Is the Clinical Congress an Unmixed Blessing?" Jones repeated this attack on the congresses in the next issue of the *California State Journal of Medicine*. See P. M. Jones, "Congress of Surgeons."

61 These worries about the knock-on effect of standardization were not unique to medicine: indeed, similar discussions were occurring in the area of educational reform around the same period, which were, in turn, fed by concerns reflected in the muckraking literature about what democracy entailed or required of a self-consciously democratic nation. See, e.g., M. R. Harris, *Five Counterrevolutionaries in Higher Education*.
62 Grimm, "Notebooks," reel 32/8-9.
63 Finney, "The Standardization of the Surgeon," 1437.
64 Grimm, "Notebooks," reel 32/8-9.
65 "Editorial: The College of Surgeons," 91. See also Young, "On the Economics of New Medical Titles," 660.
66 Codman, *The Shoulder*. See also Gainty, "The Autobiographical *Shoulder* of Ernest Amory Codman."
67 Codman, *The Shoulder*, xiii.
68 Codman, *The* Shoulder, xiii.
69 Franklin Martin offered this organic account repeatedly to medical communities. See, e.g., F. Martin, "The American College of Surgeons and Better Hospitals," 2.
70 The Carnegie Foundation had been initially uninterested in the project, but the first director of the College, John Bowman, who was also the secretary of the Carnegie Foundation, drew on his friendship with foundation president Henry Pritchett to secure the funds. L. Davis, *Fellowship of Surgeons*, 176.
71 F. Martin, "The American College of Surgeons and Better Hospitals," 2.
72 Grimm, "Notebooks," reel 32/13.
73 As the *New England Journal of Medicine* summarized the origins of the College's hospital standardization program in 1928: the "individual demand for case records" and the finding that these were "if not altogether wanting . . . fragmentary and incomplete" was the "initial incentive to the hospital standardization movement" ("The American College of Surgeons," 690).
74 Executive Committee Meeting Minutes, October 9, 1933, 46-47.
75 F. Martin, "The American College of Surgeons and Better Hospitals," 2.
76 Moulinier, "The Standardization Program of the American College of Surgeons," 11.
77 John Bowman, the first director of the College, intones this phrase in his description of the hospital standardization program origins. See, e.g., Bowman, "Case Records and Their Uses."
78 "Standard of Efficiency." By the following year, this had expanded to include additional standards for the organization of the staff, though these standards too were minimally invasive and centered mostly on the requirement that the staff be restricted to competent physicians and meet at least monthly. See "Hospital Standardization Conference."
79 Slobe, "The Hospital Survey of the College in 1921."
80 "Program of Activity," 11. See also L. Davis, *Fellowship of Surgeons*, 220-21.
81 "Hospital Betterment in California." See also "Editorial: The Annual Secretarial Conference at Chicago."
82 *Modern Times*, directed by Charlie Chaplin (United Artists, 1936).
83 See, e.g., Duffield, "The Hospital Surgeon." ACS spokesperson John Bowman addressed this kind of critique in "The Standardization of Hospitals."

84 Gamble, *Making a Place for Ourselves*, 3–34.
85 Gamble, *Making a Place for Ourselves*, 45.
86 Green, "President's Address," 17.
87 Green, "President's Address," 17.
88 A. B. Jackson, "Hospitals and Health," 118.
89 Vanessa Northington Gamble offers a very full description of the pressure standardization put on the Black hospitals in *Making a Place for Ourselves*, 35–69. See also her more concise discussion in Gamble, "The Negro Hospital Renaissance."
90 Green describes the situation in his 1922 "Annual Address of the President," 216–17, and then offers fuller details from surveys done over the intervening years regarding the hospital situation in his 1928 "President's Address," 16–17.
91 A. B. Jackson, "Hospitals and Health," 116.
92 Gamble, "The Negro Hospital Renaissance."
93 Gamble, *Making a Place for Ourselves*, 35–69, 183–85.
94 Gamble, *Making a Place for Ourselves*, 36–40.
95 Green, "Annual Address of the President," 215–16.
96 Robert Baker offers a useful and quick primer on the history of the AMA and race over the late nineteenth and early twentieth centuries. See Baker, "The American Medical Association and Race."
97 Green, "Annual Address of the President," 216.
98 Kenney, "Why a National Hospital Association?," 138.
99 National Medical Association, "Historical Manifesto."
100 For a fuller description of Washington's ideas, see chapter 4. See also, e.g., Washington, *Industrial Education for the Negro*.
101 Gamble, *Making a Place for Ourselves*, 42.
102 Kenney, "The Negro Hospital Renaissance." This issue is discussed extensively in Gamble, "The Negro Hospital Renaissance," and *Making a Place for Ourselves*, 41–42.
103 Todd Savitt makes clear that philanthropic funding was both limited and quite specifically targeted. Savitt, *Race and Medicine*, 224–36.
104 Gamble, *Making a Place for Ourselves*, 184.
105 Gamble, *Making a Place for Ourselves*, 184–88.
106 Gamble, *Making a Place for Ourselves*, 184–86.

4. THE LABOR

1 Flexner, *A Modern College and a Modern School*, 89–142.
2 Fox, "Abraham Flexner's Unpublished Report."
3 See E. R. Brown, *Rockefeller Medicine Men*. See also Flexner, *I Remember*.
4 Pritchett and Franks, *Fifth Annual Report*.
5 Pomeroy, "1910: The Year American Medicine Changed Forever," is typical of the celebratory genre in the public-facing press. Within medicine, Flexner's report is often referred to as introducing the "gold standard" of biomedical research. See, e.g., Duffy, "The Flexner Report—100 Years Later," and, more critically, Rutecki, "Clinical Science after Flexner's 1910 Report on Medical Education," 51.

6   See, e.g., Hudson, "Abraham Flexner in Perspective"; Bonner, "Abraham Flexner and the Historians"; Ludmerer, *Learning to Heal*; and Starr, *The Social Transformation of American Medicine*. Howard Berliner, "New Light on the Flexner Report," described the Flexner Report as a "cul-del-sac" for historians. Lester King repeats and expands on this idea with what seems considerable ire in "The Flexner Report of 1910."
7   Especially critical of this shift is Bonner's "Abraham Flexner and the Historians," which refers readers to the still classics of this genre: E. R. Brown, *Rockefeller Medicine Men*; Berliner, "New Light on the Flexner Report"; and Markowitz and Rosner, "Doctors in Crisis." See also Weiss and Miller, "The Social Transformation of American Medical Education."
8   This sentiment is especially well expressed in Markovitz and Rosner, "Doctors in Crisis."
9   Flexner's personal story also does not comport to this view of his significance. One of nine children of Jewish immigrants, Flexner spent his early life in Louisville, Kentucky, which set him structurally on the wrong side of industrial capitalism's brand of rough justice. As Daniel Fox has suggested, it may be the case that Flexner's and his famous brother Simon's exceptional flouting of both the classism and rampant anti-Semitism of the time engendered a kind of denialism or assimilationism that found its way into the report. See Fox's discussion in "Abraham Flexner's Unpublished Report," 491.
10 These ideas suffuse Flexner's writing, but they are pointedly expressed in his "Aristocratic and Democratic Education." See also Harris, *Five Counterrevolutionaries in Higher Education*.
11 See, e.g., Bonner, "Abraham Flexner and the Historians," 9, and Fox, "Abraham Flexner's Unpublished Report," 491.
12 Brandeis, "Trusts, Efficiency, and the New Party," 14. See also Aldrich, "On the Track of Efficiency"; Lamoreaux, "The Problem of Bigness"; Cullis, "The Limits of Progressivism"; Nyland, "Taylorism, John R. Commons, and the Hoxie Report"; Tarr, "Laboratories of Democracy?"; and Adelstein, "'Islands of Conscious Power.'"
13 Brandeis, "Trusts, Efficiency, and the New Party," 14.
14 Braverman, *Labor and Monopoly Capital*.
15 See, e.g., Miller and Weiss, "Revisiting Black Medical School Extinctions"; Savitt, "Abraham Flexner and the Black Medical Schools," and Savitt, *Race and Medicine in Nineteenth- and Early-Twentieth-Century America*. See also Hartley, "The Forgotten History of Defunct Black Medical Schools"; Wright-Mendoza, "The 1910 Report That Disadvantaged Minority Doctors."
16 As in, e.g., E. R. Brown, *Rockefeller Medicine Men*; Markowitz and Rosner, "Doctors in Crisis"; Berliner, "New Light on the Flexner Report."
17 Berliner, "New Light on the Flexner Report."
18 Thomas Bonner offers a summary of this literature in "Abraham Flexner and the Historians."
19 Flexner's "Medical Education in America," which appeared in the *Atlantic*, was simply a long excerpt from his report.
20 Forbes, "Too Many Medical Schools," which quotes extensively from Flexner, *Medical Education in the United States and Canada*.
21 Flexner, *Medical Education in the United States and Canada*, 5–7.

22 E. R. Brown, *Rockefeller Medicine Men*, 63–65.
23 Flexner, *Medical Education in the United States and Canada*, 5–7.
24 Flexner, *Medical Education in the United States and Canada*, 19. One tactic took the form of "runners" who would approach a tradesperson on the way to work in the morning extolling the economic virtues of becoming a medical practitioner. And many schools accommodated the transformation of a plumber, say, into a physician by offering their courses at night—these schools scornfully referred to as the "sundown institutions"—so that those who needed to could continue to work even as they studied. John Bowman, the president of the American College of Surgeons, offers a damning account of these practices in "The Standardization of Hospitals," 283.
25 Flexner, *Medical Education in the United States and Canada*, 3.
26 Flexner, *Medical Education in the United States and Canada*, 5.
27 Flexner, *Medical Education in the United States and Canada*, 5–7.
28 Flexner, *Medical Education in the United States and Canada*, 6.
29 Forbes, "Too Many Medical Schools," 13164.
30 Flexner, *Medical Education in the United States and Canada*, 7.
31 Flexner, *Medical Education in the United States and Canada*, 7. See also Codman, *A Study in Hospital Efficiency*.
32 Flexner, *Medical Education in the United States and Canada*, 7.
33 Flexner, *I Remember*, 74. This is an oft-quoted passage. See E. R. Brown, *Rockefeller Medicine Men*, 145, and Rutkow, *Seeking the Cure*, 151, among others.
34 Fox, "Abraham Flexner's Unpublished Report," 491.
35 Markowitz and Rosner, "Doctors in Crisis."
36 Flexner, *Medical Education*, 5.
37 Easily seen, e.g., from early evaluations of the US medical colleges. See "Medical Schools of the United States," which lists the colleges now "extinct" along with reasons for their extinction.
38 "Better Laws for the Physicians," 2.
39 Flexner, *Medical Education in the United States and Canada*, 19.
40 Flexner, *Medical Education in the United States and Canada*, 21–22.
41 Flexner, *The American College*, 20–35. See also Flexner's comments on this matter, in comparison to Prussia, in "Aristocratic and Democratic Education."
42 Flexner, "Aristocratic and Democratic Education," 387.
43 Flexner, "Aristocratic and Democratic Education," 390.
44 Flexner, "Aristocratic and Democratic Education," 393.
45 Flexner, "Adjusting the College to American Life," 370.
46 Flexner, "Aristocratic and Democratic Education, 393.
47 Flexner, "Adjusting the College to American Life," 371.
48 Pritchett, "Should the Carnegie Foundation Be Suppressed?," 562–64.
49 For a particular discussion of democratic standardization, see Pritchett, "Should the Carnegie Foundation be Suppressed," 566.
50 See, e.g., S. Thomas, "Holding the Tiger."
51 Steffens, *The Shame of the Cities*.
52 Flexner's laudatory remarks about Johns Hopkins were not limited to his autobiography. See Flexner, *Medical Education in the United States and Canada*, 12.

53 This barely scratches the surface of the relationship between the muckraking style of exposé and that of Flexner. For more on the muckrakers, see especially Stanley Schulz's classic "The Morality of Politics" and the insightful discussion offered by Cecelia Tichi in *Exposés and Excess*.
54 "Oversupply of Medical Graduates," 270. Quoted in Markowitz and Rosner, "Doctors in Crisis." 90.
55 Markowitz and Rosner, "Doctors in Crisis."
56 William Trufant Foster is probably the best known proponent of this view. See, e.g., Foster, "Planning in a Free Country," and "Dollars, Doctors, and Disease." See also Foster and Catchings, *Business without a Buyer*, which expands on these views.
57 Markowitz and Rosner, "Doctors in Crisis."
58 Flexner, *Medical Education in the United States and Canada*, 14.
59 Flexner, *Medical Education in the United States and Canada*, 14.
60 C. H. Reed, "Why Is the Profession Poor in Purse?," 975; this episode is further described in Markowitz and Rosner, "Doctors in Crisis."
61 Lydston, "Medicine as a Business Proposition." See also Lynn, "The Crime of the Century," 5.
62 Flexner mentored Lewis Mayers and Leonard V. Harrison, his colleagues at the Rockefeller Foundation's General Education Board, in a follow-up study on physician distribution in 1924. The results suggest that stabilizing physician income was critical to the rational distribution of physicians. See Mayers and Harrison, *The Distribution of Physicians in the United States*, and Daniel Fox's useful description of the study in Fox, "Abraham Flexner's Unpublished Report," 490–91.
63 Flexner, "Adjusting the College to American Life."
64 "Mr. Bynum on the Currency," 2.
65 See, e.g., the influential analysis by Paul Starr, especially *The Social Transformation of American Medicine*.
66 Berliner discusses the AMA and Carnegie Foundation responses in "New Light on the Flexner Report," 606–7.
67 "Medical Trust Makes Fight," 8.
68 Flexner, *Medical Education in the United States and Canada*, 43.
69 "Men and Things," 505.
70 "Men and Things," 505.
71 Markowitz and Rosner, "Doctors in Crisis." See also H. E. Lewis, "Editorial: Weak Medical Schools as Nurseries of Medical Genius."
72 Pritchett, "Weak Medical Schools as Nurseries of Medical Genius." See also the response of H. E. Lewis, "Editorial: Weak Medical Schools as Nurseries of Medical Genius."
73 Flexner, *Medical Education in the United States and Canada*, 43.
74 This was a finding that Flexner himself was well aware of by the 1920s. See Mayers and Harrison, *The Distribution of Physicians in the United States*.
75 "A Physician: The Plight of the Family Doctor," 7. This 1923 *New York Times* piece was reprinted in the *California State Journal of Medicine*, 21, no. 10 (1923): 449–50.
76 Bonner, "Abraham Flexner and the Historians," 3–4.
77 Savitt, *Race and Medicine*.

78   Flexner, *Medical Education in the United States and Canada*, 180.
79   Miller and Weiss, "Revisiting Black Medical School Extinctions in the Flexner Era."
80   Savitt, "Entering a White Profession." See also Du Bois, *The Philadelphia Negro*, 345–48, for his description of the "paradoxical[ly]" negative responses among the Black population to the "innovation" of Black medical practitioners.
81   See, e.g., Washington, *Industrial Education for the Negro*, and Du Bois, "The Talented Tenth."
82   Savitt's detailed account of the Black medical schools of this era, which traces also the fates of students trained there, nicely illustrates the reductive nature of Flexner's analyses. See Savitt, *Race and Medicine* and "Abraham Flexner and the Black Medical Schools."
83   Interested readers can find the "Salt Wagon Story" on the "Mission and Vision" page of the Meharry Medical College website, accessed March 2, 2024, https://home.mmc.edu/about/mission-vision/.
84   Flexner, *Medical Education in the United States and Canada*, 180.
85   Thirkield to Pritchett, February 21, 1910. See also Savitt's further discussion of Thirkield's appeals to the Carnegie and then Rockefeller Foundations in *Race and Medicine*, 224–36.
86   Savitt, *Race and Medicine*, 224–36.
87   Du Bois, *The Philadelphia Negro*, 354.
88   Savitt, *Race and Medicine*, 238–60.
89   Flexner to Pritchett, April 27, 1921.
90   Flexner to Pritchett, April 27, 1921.

5. THE MARKET

1   "Today in Tucson."
2   Strasser, "Sponsorship and Snake Oil," 101.
3   Nany Tomes offers wonderful descriptions of these campaigns in *The Gospel of Germs* and in "Epidemic Entertainments." See also Abrams, "'Spitting Is Dangerous, Indecent, and against the Law,'" and Rogers, "Germs with Legs."
4   "Surgeons Open Sectional Meet in City Today."
5   "Distinguished Surgeons Gather in Health Rally at Tucson High School."
6   "Distinguished Surgeons Gather in Health Rally." See also Program of the Community Health Meeting, Wednesday, October 11, 1933.
7   See, e.g., the descriptions of educational campaigns in Ostherr, *Medical Visions*. See also Posner, "Communicating Disease," and Ostherr, "Medical Education through Film."
8   Grimm, "Notebooks," reel 32/9. See also Moulinier, "Hospital Standardization and the Medical and Nursing Professions," 30.
9   For an interesting and contemporaneous discussion of standardization and mass production more generally, see Kyrk, *A Theory of Consumption*.
10   The classic here is undoubtedly Cowan, *More Work for Mother*.
11   Moulinier in a discussion of Kanavel, "The Hospital as an Educational Center," 44.
12   "German Armies Turn West toward Paris, Gain Six Miles. Do Not Cross the Marne; Fighting Rages Fiercely near Soissons," *New York Times*, June 2, 1918.

13 Bowman, "Best of Care for Every Hospital Patient," 2.
14 Bowman, "Best of Care for Every Hospital Patient," 2.
15 Bowman, "Best of Care for Every Hospital Patient," 13.
16 Hawthorne, "Better Hospitals for Everybody," 202.
17 Hawthorne, "Better Hospitals for Everybody," 203.
18 Hawthorne, "Better Hospitals for Everybody," 208.
19 Forbes, "Too Many Medical Schools."
20 "Oregon Surgeons to Meet on Friday for Conference."
21 "American College of Surgeons Admits 756 to Fellowship."
22 P. M. Jones, "The Costume of the College."
23 "An Unusual Meeting at the New City Auditorium," *Daily Clarion Ledger*, Jackson, Mississippi, January 25, 1924.
24 Moulinier, "Hospital Standardization and the Medical and Nursing Professions," 30.
25 Dunott, "Report of Recommendations of the American Railway Association." See also "Local Hospital Given Approval."
26 "Vital Importance Child Welfare Work Urged in Rousing Addresses at Community Health Gathering."
27 "Surgeons Here Stack Up with Best—Franklin."
28 "Community Health Meeting Features 2-Day Convention of College of Surgeons."
29 "Dr. Brady's Health Talks: Some Surgeons Are Poor Waiters." This article also appeared on May 7, 1933, in the *Brooklyn Daily Eagle* under the title "Brass Surgeons or Piker Doctors?"
30 In 1924, the circulated text read in part: "The movement aims directly at the elimination of deficiencies in hospital services to the patient and the establishment of closer supervision and checkup on the work of the institution. It has been rapid in its acceptance and accomplishment, because of the whole-hearted co-operation of the hospital people and public generally, of the United States and Canada." See, e.g., "Surgeons Make a Hospital Survey" and "Our Hospitals Work for Human Salvage." The same story, albeit with different local details, ran in many locations; see, in addition, e.g., the *Newark Advocate* on October 13, 1930, and the *Bangor Daily News* on October 20, 1930.
31 Board of Regents Meeting Minutes, October 17, 1932. Writes Edward McCormick of Malcolm MacEachern, upon his retirement from the College in 1950, "If, in the popular parlance of today, anybody should ever attempt a 'Mr. Hospital' he most certainly would have to select one person and one alone—Dr. MacEachern." See McCormick, "Dr. Malcolm T. MacEachern Retires," 24.
32 "Patients Watched after Discharge."
33 State Executive Committee Meeting, October 24, 1922.
34 Board of Regents Meeting Minutes, October 17, 1932.
35 Executive Committee Meeting Minutes, June 10, 1934, III-12.
36 Executive Committee Meeting Minutes, June 10, 1934, III-12.
37 Executive Committee Meeting Minutes, June 10, 1934, III-12.
38 "Physicians to Give Series of Talks."
39 Radio Programs listed by the Meriden (CT) *Record-Journal*, October 10, 1933.
40 Browy, "Dogs Suffer No Pain in Experiment."

41 See, e.g., "A Physician: The Plight of the Family Doctor."
42 "Better Cooperation between Public and Surgeons Is Plea Made at Medical Convention."
43 "Public Service Aim of Doctors' Society."
44 Though the term *silent majority* was for a long time a euphemism for the dead, during the early twentieth century, and particularly around the candidacy of Calvin Coolidge—whose best characteristic, according to Sinclair Lewis's *The Man Who Knew Coolidge*, was that he was "SAFE"—its use shifted to reflect what a *Collier's* journalist described as "the great majority of Americans" who were "neither radicals nor reactionaries" but instead "middle-of-the road folks who own their own homes and work hard, and would like to have the government get back to its old habits of meddling with their lives as little as possible." See Barton, "Concerning Calvin Coolidge," 8, also quoted and further discussed in Kerry Buckley's excellent "A President for the 'Great Silent Majority.'"
45 From 1923 onward, the College began to embrace film as a useful channel of public engagement, so much so that by 1926, it was cooperating with Will Hays, the president of the Motion Picture Producers and Distributors of America and author of the famously puritanical motion picture production code of 1930. The Hays Code policed Hollywood; the College policed medical filmmaking. See, e.g., "Movies Enter New Field of Science Today." Will Hays attended the October 1926 convention in which the medical motion picture collaboration was conceived. See also Hays, "Medical Motion Pictures," a laudatory speech delivered to the Meeting of the Board of Governors and Fellows on October 15, 1931.
46 "Angry Cleric Calls Vaccine Filthy Poison."
47 State Executive Committee Meeting, October 24, 1922.
48 See, e.g., "Vital Importance Child Welfare Work."
49 "Vital Importance of Early Medical Attention Stressed at Surgeons' Mass Meeting."
50 "Better Cooperation between Public and Surgeons Is Plea Made at Medical Convention."
51 "Public Service Aim of Doctors' Society." See also, e.g., "Surgeons Spend Busy Day Here"; "Wild Youth Warned to Check Fast Pace"; Mavity, "Surgeons at S. F. Congress to Banish Fear of Knife at Mass Meeting Tonight."
52 "Wild Youth Warned to Check Fast Pace."
53 "Lincoln Hears Doctors."
54 "Public Service Aim of Doctors' Society."
55 "More Care of Health Urged by College of Surgeons Public Meeting Here Monday."
56 "Distinguished Surgeons Gather in Health Rally." See also Program of the Community Health Meeting, Wednesday, October 11, 1933.
57 "Distinguished Surgeons Gather in Health Rally."
58 "Medical Science Beating Disease, Statistics Show."
59 Ator, "Doctor Applies Stethoscope to New Deal in US."
60 Von Neupert, "Dr. Carl von Neupert Discusses American College of Surgeons."
61 Though not discussed with great regularity, some noted that the medical situation for the Black communities in the South and for immigrant communities scattered

throughout the country remained essentially unchanged. See, e.g., M. Davis, "Problems of Health Service for Negroes," and Dublin, *Health and Wealth*.
62 Ator, "Doctor Applies Stethoscope to New Deal in US."
63 "Dr. Mayo Hails New Drive on Germs."
64 "Deformed Boy and Girl Aid Science and Selves."
65 "Surgeons Perform Miracle of Science."
66 "Big Outdoor Meeting Set for Sunday."
67 Executive Committee Meeting Minutes, October 9, 1933.
68 "US Hospitals for Veterans Are Attacked"; "Charges Relief Patients Burden US Hospitals"; "Public Support Urged to Save Voluntary Hospitals."
69 "Free Clinics Damage to Doctors Says Fr. Brennan."
70 See, e.g., Laurence, "Health Insurance Gets Official Aid," which is a summary of the College's position that appeared in the *New York Times* in 1934.

6. MONOPOLY

1 "Here's Text of Board's Report on Hospital"; "Lid off in Hospital Row."
2 "Here's Text of Board's Report on Hospital."
3 "Here's Text of Board's Report on Hospital."
4 "Sprinkle Out as Head Man; Bar 9 Doctors from Staff."
5 "Here's Text of Board's Report on Hospital."
6 "Sprinkle Out as Head Man; Bar 9 Doctors from Staff."
7 "Here's Text of Board's Report on Hospital."
8 Despite the synchronous condemnations of the Tampa hospital, it was the AMA, and not the ACS or AHA, that was adamantly against any reimbursement relationship other than a fee-for-service arrangement. As early as 1934, the ACS had explicitly broken with the AMA on the matter, suggesting publicly that the only way to make health care affordable for the "citizen of average means" was to introduce a system of voluntary prepayment at the community level; Laurence, "To Urge Reduction in Hospital Costs."
9 Wright, "Taylorism Reconsidered." See also Braverman, *Labor and Monopoly Capital*; Clawson, *Bureaucracy and the Labor Process*, 31–33; Merkle, *Management and Ideology*; Kelly, *Scientific Management, Job Redesign and Work Performance*; Meiksins, "Scientific Management and Class Relations"; Nyland, "Scientific Management and Planning"; Nyland, *Reduced Worktime and the Management of Production*.
10 "The American Medical Association Decision."
11 See especially Morris Fishbein's views here as described in, e.g., "Health Systems Decried." Stefan Link has described the populist vibe that guided much of the industrial capitalism of the early twentieth century. Though he limits his purview just to the Fordist tradition, his observations fit well with the aims and goals of industrial efficiency more broadly. See Link, *Forging Global Fordism*, 1–50.
12 Chris Wright has a useful discussion in his "Taylorism Reconsidered." Though it considers the Australian workplace, the historiographical trajectory of Taylorism is well laid out. See also Stefan Link on Fordism. Though Link recovers Fordism from the totalizing traditions it had fallen into, he continues to see Taylorism according

to the traditions set out for its discussion in the 1970s. See Link, *Forging Global Fordism*, 1–18.

13 This concept is traced briefly in Gainty, "Why Wait?"
14 Nancy Tomes's work on the history of consumerism in medicine offers a refreshing pushback against this view, noting that although "this view of medicine as a special market case reflects the unique position that the doctor-patient relationship came to occupy (and still occupies) in the world of twentieth-century goods and services," there is good reason to think that "scholars have overstated medicine's exception from the currents of modern consumerism," not least because "the conception of medical goods and services as 'special' depended on comparing them with other categories of goods and services" in the first place; Tomes, "Merchants of Health," 545. See also Tomes, *Remaking the American Patient*, for further details and a more expansive discussion.
15 Ameringer, *The Health Care Revolution*, 32. The literature on this moment of medical monopoly is voluminous, with the preponderance written in the late 1970s–1980s period. See, e.g., Ward, "United States versus American Medical Association et al."; Starr, *The Social Transformation*; Tomes, *Remaking the American Patient*; Rosenberg, *The Care of Strangers*; Stevens, *In Sickness and in Wealth*; Rosen, "Contract or Lodge Practice and Its Influence on Medical Attitudes to Health Insurance"; Anderson, *Health Services in the United States*; Burrow, AMA: *Voice of American Medicine*, and *Organized Medicine in the Progressive Era*; Rayack, *Professional Power and American Medicine*; Hirshfield, *The Lost Reform*; Weller, "'Free Choice' as a Restraint of Trade," and "Antitrust Joint Ventures and the End of the AMA's Contract Practice Ethics"; Fox, *Health Policies, Health Politics*.
16 Garceau, "Organized Medicine Enforces Its 'Party Line,'" 419. See also Garceau, *The Political Life of the American Medical Association*.
17 Garceau, "Organized Medicine Enforces Its 'Party Line,'" 418.
18 Rorty, *American Medicine Mobilizes*, 140–46. Michael Shadid describes this situation in his multiple texts. See Shadid, *A Doctor for the People*, and *Doctors of Today and Tomorrow*. See also Kessel, "Price Discrimination in Medicine." Rosemary Stevens's description in *American Medicine and the Public Interest* (188) and Paul Starr's in *The Social Transformation* (303–4) are exemplary of the medical historical view.
19 Shadid, *A Doctor for the People*. This story is also well described in Kessel, "Price Discrimination in Medicine," 20–53.
20 Rorty, *American Medicine Mobilizes*, 117.
21 Rorty, *American Medicine Mobilizes*, 127. See also Tomes, *Remaking the American Patient*, 123.
22 Davis, *America Organizes Medicine*. See also Waldemar Kaempffert's review of the book in the same year: "Speaking of Doctors and How They Take Care of You: A Thorough and Objective Study of Medical Care in America by Michael Davis."
23 The stalwart defender of prepayment systems and group practice, Hugh Cabot, said in a speech to the Group Health Association in Washington, DC, on May 5, 1938, that the AMA's claims to "'sole control of medical practice'" was "'pure fascism of the Italian type.'" It was that quote that earned him a headline in the same day's *New York Times*, which read "Assails Fascism in Medical Field: Dr. Cabot of Mayo Clinic Hits 'Organized Medicine' in Talk to Health Association." Of course, the AMA viewed Cabot as part of its socialist opposition.

24 Fishbein, "The Report of the Committee on the Costs of Medical Care," 2034–35. See also Tomes, *Remaking the American Patient* (73–76) for a useful discussion of these terms and their purpose.
25 This is well explained by Weller, "'Free Choice' as a Restraint of Trade," 1366. Weller quotes here from the Bureau of Medical Economics, American Medical Association, *Group Hospitalization*, 39–40.
26 See, e.g., Weller, "'Free Choice' as a Restraint of Trade."
27 Goldwater, "Dispensaries," 615.
28 Beito, *From Mutual Aid to the Welfare State*, 25–45.
29 M. Davis, "Problems of Health Services for Negroes," 440–41.
30 See, e.g., Thorning, "Social Medicine in Cuba," whose work on cooperative health care organizations was discussed in the US Congress in relation to health reform taking place during the 1940s. For a fuller picture of the Ybor social clubs generally, see Long, "An Immigrant Co-Operative Medicine Program in the South," and Mormino and Pozzetta, *The Immigrant World of Ybor City*.
31 Mormino and Pozzetta, *The Immigrant World of Ybor City*, 198.
32 Mormino and Pozzetta, *The Immigrant World of Ybor City*, 197–205.
33 See, e.g., Burrow, *Organized Medicine in the Progressive Era*; Fox, *Health Policies, Health Politics*; Starr, *The Social Transformation*; and Stevens, *In Sickness and in Wealth*.
34 Patricia Spain Ward offers a clear and cogent discussion of the case itself in "United States versus American Medical Association et al." See also Raub, "The Anti-Trust Prosecution against the American Medical Association."
35 "Monopoly Move Hailed by G.H.A."
36 "Action to Set Up New Health Unit Here Is Deferred."
37 See, e.g., Ward, "United States versus American Medical Association et al."
38 Paul Starr's explanation of this phenomenon is exemplary; Starr, *The Social Transformation*, 198–234 and 300–305.
39 Foster, "Dollars, Doctors, and Disease." See also Foster, "Planning in a Free Country."
40 See, e.g., Filene, "The Minimum Wage and Efficiency"; Brookings, *The Way Forward*; Leven, Moulton, and Warburton, *America's Capacity to Consume*; Foster and Catchings, *Business without a Buyer*; Tugwell, *Industry's Coming of Age*.
41 Beaudreau and Taylor, "Why Did the Roosevelt Administration Think Cartels, Higher Wages, and Shorter Workweeks Would Promote Recovery from the Great Depression?"
42 This is a very brief overview of a very complex situation. In addition to Beaudreau and Taylor's useful summary work, "Why Did the Roosevelt Administration," see also Field, *A Great Leap Forward*; O'Brien, Taylor, and Selgin, "By Our Bootstraps"; and O'Brien, "A Behavioral Explanation for Nominal Wage Rigidity during the Great Depression."
43 There is much debate, however, on what the NIRA actually accomplished. See the useful summary in Hannsgen and Papadimitriou, "Did the New Deal Prolong or Worsen the Great Depression?"
44 Weller, "'Free Choice' as a Restraint of Trade," 1355, quoting the Bureau of Medical Economics, American Medical Association, *An Introduction to Medical Economics*.

45 Ameringer, *The Health Care Revolution*, 32. Carl Ameringer draws heavily from Wells, *Antitrust and the Formation of the Postwar World*.
46 Charles Weller gives especially good evidence that the AMA understood NIRA as a prompt for it to open up the floodgates of the coercive behavior for which it became known. See Weller, "'Free Choice' as a Restraint of Trade," 1355. The Supreme Court found NIRA unconstitutional in the 1935 decision *A.L.A. Schechter Poultry Corporation v. United States*.
47 Ameringer, *The Health Care Revolution*, 32–35.
48 See, e.g., Shryock, "Freedom and Interference in Medicine," and Committee on the Cost of Medical Care, *Medical Care for the American People*, 3.
49 Ameringer, *The Health Care Revolution*, 35, quoting *United States v. American Medical Association et al.*
50 *American Medical Association v. United States*.
51 Ameringer, *The Health Care Revolution*, 34–37. As Ameringer notes, the court case was already uniquely situated since the precipitating events had taken place in Washington, DC. Since DC is not a state, Arnold did not have to consider the sticky requirements of the Constitution's commerce clause, which restricted federal authority to commerce between the states. The AMA's actions elsewhere would be much harder to police.
52 Brandeis, "Trusts, Efficiency, and the New Party." Brandeis describes the purchase of Andrew Carnegie's US Steel, in the formation of the Steel Trust, as an example of the desire of monopolies to preserve *inefficiency* in the market. US Steel had been so efficient that no company could come near its prices. "Because his competitors were unable to rise to his remarkable efficiency, his business career was killed; and the American people were deprived of his ability—his genius—to produce steel cheaply." For more on Brandeis's views, see Aldrich, "On the Track of Efficiency"; Lamoreaux, "The Problem of Bigness"; Cullis, "The Limits of Progressivism"; Nyland, "Taylorism, John R. Commons, and the Hoxie Report"; Tarr, "Laboratories of Democracy?"; Adelstein, "'Islands of Conscious Power.'"
53 Ameringer, *The Health Care Revolution*, 34.
54 Arnold, *Voltaire and the Cowboy*, 462–63. See also discussions in Ameringer, *The Health Care Revolution*, 32–34, and Wells, *Antitrust and the Formation of the Postwar World*.
55 *American Medical Association v. United States*. Fishbein is quoted in Ward, "United States versus American Medical Association et al.," 144.
56 The College was dedicated to some form of prepayment and in this way found itself on the wrong side of the AMA.
57 Committee on the Cost of Medical Care, *Medical Care for the American People*, 3.
58 See, e.g., "Doctors Denounced," as well as the book it describes: Barnesby, *Medical Chaos and Crime*.
59 Hugh Cabot at the National Health Conference, July 18–21, 1938. Quoted in Rorty, *American Medicine Mobilizes*, 34. For the sect supposedly most closely allied with science, the decided dearth of scientifically inflected medical change over the early twentieth century was a worry. Medicine had improved dramatically over the tail end of the nineteenth century, yet by the time the most lauded features of medicine appeared, it had fallen into a period of relative stasis, worried some within the

profession, with far fewer dramatic improvements. There still wasn't much in their healing arsenals that could address the major causes of death and debility, which offered reason to suspect that the allopathic mode had stalled. It was a view somewhat allayed by the introduction of sulfa drugs and then antibiotics over the late 1930s and 1940s. But in the 1950s, similar concerns over whether medical science had actually improved the care of health arose once more, this time in the form of consternation over whether downward trends in mortality related to infectious disease could actually be attributed to medical interventions. See, e.g., Magill, "The Immunologist and the Evil Spirits"; McKeown and Record, "Medical Evidence Related to English Population Changes in the Eighteenth Century"; McKeown and Record, "Reasons for the Decline of Mortality in England and Wales during the Nineteenth Century." Those working in the other medical sects, still not totally gone by the 1930s, thought that the lack of evidence for allopathic medicine's effectiveness ought to be called more sharply to attention. See, e.g., Peterkin, "Ethical Economics."

60 Vanessa Northington Gamble offers a striking example of what federal provision for the care of Black veterans looked like in the interwar period in her discussion of the Tuskegee Veterans Hospital in Alabama, which, as one critic pointed out, was "in the lynching belt" of the South (Gamble, *Making a Place for Ourselves*, 78). In this same text, Gamble points that integration as a policy for hospitals really only came to be on the agenda after World War II.

61 Committee on the Cost of Medical Care, *Medical Care for the American People*, 14–15.

62 Given how relatively inexpensive these medical providers and their products were, these figures indicate that a not insignificant portion of the population continued to rely partially or wholly on these services. The presence of this recalcitrant population segment explained another one of the shared sentiments among health's bickering elites that whatever else was true, the average person needed to be further "educated" to make "better" medical choices. This was another of the few areas in which the authors of the CCMC minority report expressed their "hearty" agreement with the majority view, even as, to nearly all other points, they took great offense. Committee on the Cost of Medical Care, *Medical Care for the American People*, 14–15.

63 Shryock, "Freedom and Interference in Medicine," 49. See also "The Achilles Heel of American Medicine," 360.

64 Sigerist, *Medicine and Human Welfare*, 139. Also quoted in Rorty, *American Medicine Mobilizes*, 87.

65 See Pooley, "James Rorty's Voice," and Rorty, *Our Master's Voice*.

66 Orr, "Review: *American Medicine Mobilizes*." See also Barker, "Review: *American Medicine Mobilizes*."

67 Garceau, "Organized Medicine Enforces Its 'Party Line,'" and *Political Life of the American Medical Association*.

68 Nancy Tomes offers a compelling and full description in *Remaking the American Patient*, 105–38.

69 "The American Medical Association," 91.

70 "The American Medical Association," 92; see also Kaempffert, "Diagnosing the Case of Organized Medicine Today."

71 Bernheim, *Medicine at the Crossroads*.

72 Garceau, "Organized Medicine Enforces its 'Party Line,'" 415.
73 Garceau, "Organized Medicine Enforces its 'Party Line,'" 415.
74 "The American Medical Association," 90–91.
75 Barker, "Review: *American Medicine Mobilizes*," 580. Creighton Barker describes with distaste Rorty's depiction of Morris Fishbein as a "villain in false whiskers" and his "nominat[ion] of Isadore Falk for a halo."
76 Fishbein, "The Report of the Committee on the Costs of Medical Care," 2035. See also Committee on the Cost of Medical Care, *Medical Care for the American People*, 153–54.
77 Wright, "Taylorism Reconsidered," 35.
78 This conflation of government and big business was consistent in many ways with the rhetoric of those explicitly antagonistic to the incursions of the federal government to intervene in the hospital sector around the question of veteran health services. Incensed at what was taken to be unfair competition, an outraged Robert Jolly, president of the American Hospital Association in 1935, argued that the government "has no more business going into competition with the hospital business than with any other business" ("US Hospitals for Veterans Are Attacked"). See also, e.g., "Charges Relief Patients Burden US Hospitals."
79 Fishbein, "The Report of the Committee on the Costs of Medical Care," 2035.
80 Committee on the Cost of Medical Care, *Medical Care for the American People*, 39–40.
81 Fishbein, "The Committee on the Costs of Medical Care," 1950.
82 "Medical Leaders Organize to Fight Destructive Propaganda."
83 Warner, "The Aesthetic Grounding of Modern Medicine," 32–45.
84 "Assails Fascism in Medical Field."
85 Laurence, "Nation's Doctors Called to Revolt" *New York Times* April 7, 1938, 1, 24.
86 E. Jackson, "Letter to the Editor: Doctor and Patient," 1386.

AFTERWORD

1 Cochrane, *Effectiveness and Efficiency*, 4–5.
2 Frank Jones, "British Doctor Says Medicine Has Become Too Elaborate," *Toronto Star*, March 22, 1972, box ALC/5/1-ALC/5/3, Archives of Archie Cochrane, Library Special Collections, University of Cardiff, Cardiff, Wales.
3 Cochrane retells this story quite often; this version is taken from a TV broadcast. See BBC TV, "The Trouble with Medicine."
4 Donabedian, "The End Results of Health Care," 233.
5 Codman, *The Shoulder*, xxxviii.
6 Though McKeown laid this out over a number of different publications, perhaps the most accessible summary is contained in his book *The Role of Medicine*.
7 Magill, "The Immunologist and the Evil Spirits."
8 See Illich, *Medical Nemesis*, 165. Illich made his comments about his disinterest in medicine in the preface to a later 1995 edition, newly titled *Limits to Medicine*. For a brief but effective discussion of both works together, see Bunker, "Ivan Illich and Medical Nemesis."
9 See, e.g., Freidson, *Profession of Medicine*, and Starr, *The Social Transformation*.
10 E. R. Brown, *Rockefeller Medicine Men*.

11 Reverby and Rosner, "Beyond 'the Great Doctors.'"
12 Sarah Palin, "Statement on the Current Health Care Debate," *Facebook*, August 7, 2009.
13 See, e.g., Frankford, "The Remarkable Staying Power of 'Death Panels.'"
14 Shortliffe, "The Adolescence of AI in Medicine," 93.
15 The news was everywhere, and it was partly an advertising ploy to draw attention to the new genetically focused pharmaceutical research at GlaxoSmithKline that was supposed to correct this problem by producing more personalized drugs. See, e.g., Connor, "Glaxo Chief."

Bibliography

Abrams, Jeanne. "'Spitting Is Dangerous, Indecent, and against the Law!' Legislating Health Behavior during the American Tuberculosis Crusade." *Journal of the History of Medicine and Allied Sciences* 68, no. 3 (2013): 416-50.
"Achilles Heel of American Medicine, The." *California and Western Medicine* 51, no. 6 (1939): 360-62.
"Action to Set Up New Health Unit Here Is Deferred." *Washington Evening Star*, December 3, 1937.
Adams, Annemarie. *Medicine by Design: The Architect and the Modern Hospital, 1893-1943*. Minneapolis: University of Minnesota Press, 2008.
Adams, Luther. "Review: Beth Tompkins Bates, *The Making of Black Detroit in the Age of Henry Ford*." *Business History Review* 88, no. 3 (2014): 615-17.
Adelstein, Richard P. "'Islands of Conscious Power': Louis D. Brandeis and the Modern Corporation." *Business History Review* 63, no. 3 (1989): 614-56.
Ahuja, Nitin. "Fordism in the Hospital." *Journal of the History of Medicine and Allied Sciences* 67, no. 3 (2012): 398-427.
Aitken, Hugh. *Scientific Management in Action: Taylorism at Watertown Arsenal, 1908-1915*. Cambridge, MA: Harvard University Press, 1960.
A. L. A. Schechter Poultry Corporation v. United States, 295 US 495 (1935).
Aldrich, Mark. "On the Track of Efficiency: Scientific Management Comes to Railroad Shops, 1900-1930." *Business History Review* 84, no. 3 (2010): 501-26.
Alexander, Jennifer Karns. *The Mantra of Efficiency: From Waterwheel to Social Control*. Baltimore: Johns Hopkins University Press, 2008.
"American College of Surgeons, The." *New England Journal of Medicine* 199, no. 14 (1928): 690.
"American College of Surgeons Admits 756 to Fellowship." *Boston Globe*, October 28, 1922.
"American Medical Association, The." *Fortune* 18, no. 5 (1938): 88-92, 150, 152, 156, 158, 160, 162, 164, 166, 168.
"American Medical Association Decision, The." *Hawaii Tribune-Herald*, January 19, 1943.
American Medical Association v. United States, 317 US 519 (1943).

Ameringer, Carl. *The Health Care Revolution: From Medical Monopoly to Market Competition*. Berkeley: University of California Press, 2008.

Anderson, Odin. *Health Services in the United States: A Growth Enterprise since 1875*. Ann Arbor: University of Michigan Press, 1985.

"Angry Cleric Calls Vaccine Filthy Poison." *Hartford Courant*, March 2, 1927.

Antonio, Robert, and Alessandro Bonnano. "A New Global Capitalism? From 'Americanism and Fordism' to 'Americanization-Globalization.'" *American Studies* 41, no. 2/3 (2000): 33–77.

"Appendectomy," February 23, 1915, MSP 8, box 55, folder 5, Frank and Lillian Gilbreth Library of Management Research and Professional Papers, Purdue University Archives and Special Collections, West Lafayette, IN.

Arnold, Thurman W. *Voltaire and the Cowboy: The Letters of Thurman Arnold*, edited by Gene Gressley. Boulder: Colorado Associated University Press, 1977.

"Assails Fascism in Medical Field: Dr. Cabot of Mayo Clinic Hits 'Organized Medicine' in Talk to Health Association." *New York Times*, May 5, 1938.

Ator, Joseph. "Doctor Applies Stethoscope to New Deal in US." *Chicago Tribune*, October 10, 1933.

Babson, Roger. "What Henry Ford Really Said to Roger Babson." *The Sun*, January 24, 1915.

Baker, Robert B. "The American Medical Association and Race." *Virtual Mentor* 16, no. 6 (2014): 479–88.

Baldwin, J. F., to Frank Gilbreth, March 4, 1916, MSP 8, box 56, 0416-4, Frank and Lillian Gilbreth Library of Management Research and Professional Papers, Purdue University Archives and Special Collections, West Lafayette, IN.

Barker, Creighton. "Review: *American Medicine Mobilizes*." *Yale Journal of Biology and Medicine* 11, no. 5 (1939): 580.

Barnesby, Norman. *Medical Chaos and Crime*. New York: M. Kennerley, 1910.

Barton, Bruce. "Concerning Calvin Coolidge." *Collier's*, November 22, 1919, 8, 24, 28.

Bates, Beth Tompkins. *The Making of Black Detroit in the Age of Henry Ford*. Chapel Hill: University of North Carolina Press, 2012.

Bauch, Nicholas. "The Extensible Digestive System: Biotechnology at the Battle Creek Sanitarium, 1890–1900." *Cultural Geographies* 18, no. 2. (2011): 209–29.

Bauch, Nicholas. *A Geography of Digestion: Biotechnology and the Kellogg Cereal Enterprise*. Oakland: University of California Press, 2017.

BBC TV. "The Trouble with Medicine." Series 13, episode 21, *BBC Horizon*, July 22, 1977.

Beard, Richard Olding. "The Mayo Clinic Building, Rochester, Minnesota." *Journal-Lancet* 34, no. 16 (1914): 425–34.

Beaudreau, Bernard C., and Jason E. Taylor. "Why Did the Roosevelt Administration Think Cartels, Higher Wages, and Shorter Workweeks Would Promote Recovery from the Great Depression?" *The Independent Review* 23, no. 1 (2018): 91–107.

Beckert, Sven, Angus Burgin, Peter James Hudson, Louis Hyman, Naomi Lamoreaux, Scott Marler, Stephen Mihm, et al. "Interchange: The History of Capitalism," *Journal of American History* 101, no. 2 (2014): 503–36.

Beito, David T. *From Mutual Aid to the Welfare State: Fraternal Societies and Social Service, 1890–1967*. Chapel Hill: University of North Carolina Press, 2000.

Beniger, James R. *The Control Revolution: Technological and Economic Origins of the Information Society.* Cambridge, MA: Harvard University Press, 1986.

Berliner, Howard. "New Light on the Flexner Report: Notes on the AMA-Carnegie Foundation Background." *Bulletin of the History of Medicine* 51, no. 4. (1977): 603–9.

Berliner, Howard. *A System of Scientific Medicine: Philanthropic Foundations in the Flexner Era.* New York: Tavistock, 1986.

Bernheim, Bertram. *Medicine at the Crossroads.* New York: W. Morrow, 1939.

Berwick, Donald. "E. A. Codman and the Rhetoric of Battle: A Commentary." *Milbank Quarterly* 67 (1989): 262–67.

"Better Cooperation between Public and Surgeons Is Plea Made at Medical Convention." *Bisbee Daily Review*, November 21, 1920.

"Better Laws for the Physicians: Committee Is Named by the Homeopathic Institute to Secure Legislation." *The Times*, June 23, 1900.

"Big Outdoor Meeting Set for Sunday." *Oakland Tribune*, April 25, 1931.

Board of Regents Meeting Minutes, May 15, 1913, RG4/SG04/S02, Minutes of the Board of Regents, the Board of Governors, the Fellows, and Committees, Archives of the American College of Surgeons, Chicago, IL.

Board of Regents Meeting Minutes, October 17, 1932, RG4/SG04/S02, Minutes of the Board of Regents, the Board of Governors, the Fellows, and Committees, Archives of the American College of Surgeons, Chicago, IL.

Bonner, Thomas. "Abraham Flexner and the Historians." *Journal of the History of Medicine and Allied Sciences* 45, no. 1 (1990): 3–10.

Boston Women's Health Book Collective. *Our Bodies, Ourselves.* New York: Simon & Schuster, 1973.

Bowker, Geoffrey, and Susan Leigh Star. *Sorting Things Out: Classification and Its Consequences.* Cambridge, MA: MIT Press, 1999.

Bowman, John. "Best of Care for Every Hospital Patient." *New York Times Magazine*, June 2, 1918, 2, 13.

Bowman, John. "Case Records and Their Uses." *Bulletin of the American College of Surgeons* 4, no. 1 (1919): 1–14.

Bowman, John. "The Standardization of Hospitals." *Boston Medical and Surgical Journal* 177, no. 9 (1917): 283–84.

Brandeis, Louis. "Trusts, Efficiency, and the New Party." *Collier's Weekly*, September 14, 1912, 14–15.

Braverman, Harry. *Labor and Monopoly Capital: The Degradation of Work in the Twentieth Century.* New York: Monthly Review Press, 1974.

Brickner, Walter M. "The College of Surgeons." *American Journal of Surgery* 27, no. 6 (1913): 234–35.

Broderick, R. G. "The Effect of the Eight Hour Day on the Hospital Budget." *Modern Hospital* 16, no. 4 (1921): 337–38.

Brookings, Robert. *The Way Forward.* New York: Macmillan, 1932.

Brown, Elspeth. *The Corporate Eye: Photography and the Rationalization of American Commercial Culture.* Baltimore: Johns Hopkins University Press, 2005.

Brown, E. Richard. *Rockefeller Medicine Men: Medicine and Capitalism in America.* Berkeley: University of California Press, 1979.

Browy, Calmer. "Dogs Suffer No Pain in Experiment." *The Capital Times*, November 11, 1927.
Buckley, Kerry. "A President for the 'Great Silent Majority': Bruce Barton's Construction of Calvin Coolidge." *New England Quarterly* 76, no. 4 (2003): 593-626.
Bunker, J. P. "Ivan Illich and Medical Nemesis." *Journal of Epidemiology and Community Health (1979-)* 57, no. 12 (2003): 927.
Bureau of Medical Economics, American Medical Association. *Group Hospitalization*. Chicago: American Medical Association, 1937.
Bureau of Medical Economics, American Medical Association. *An Introduction to Medical Economics*. Chicago: American Medical Association, 1935.
Burrow, James G. AMA: *Voice of American Medicine*. Baltimore: Johns Hopkins University Press, 1963.
Burrow, James G. *Organized Medicine in the Progressive Era: The Move toward Monopoly*. Baltimore: Johns Hopkins University Press, 1977.
"Business Man's Businesslike Hospital, A." *Washington Times*, August 12, 1918.
Cabot, Richard. "Better Doctoring for Less Money." *American Magazine* 81, no. 5 (1916): 43-44, 76-78, 81.
Caton, Donald. "Who Said Childbirth Is Natural? The Medical Mission of Grantly Dick Read." *Anesthesiology* 84 (1996): 955-64.
Chandler, Alfred. *The Visible Hand. The Managerial Revolution in American Business*. Cambridge, MA: Harvard University Press, 1977.
"Charges Relief Patients Burden US Hospitals." *Chicago Tribune*, May 2, 1935.
Chenery, William L. "Ford Hospital Upsets the Old Medical Traditions." *New York Times*, August 24, 1924, 7.
Chimes, Enisse. "The History of the Henry Ford Hospital." Unpublished, n.d., ca. 1977, Series 7, Henry Ford Hospital History Research Materials, Enisse Chimes Collection, Conrad R. Lam Archives, Henry Ford Health, Detroit, MI.
Clawson, Dan. *Bureaucracy and the Labor Process: The Transformation of US Industry, 1860-1920*. New York: Monthly Review Press, 1980.
Cobley, Evelyn. *Modernism and the Culture of Efficiency: Ideology and Friction*. Toronto: University of Toronto Press, 2009.
Cochrane, Archie. *Effectiveness and Efficiency: Random Reflections on Health Services*. London: Nuffield Trust, 1972.
Code of Ethics of the American Medical Association Adopted 1847. Philadelphia: T. K. and P. G. Collins, 1854.
Codman, Ernest Amory. "The Product of a Hospital." *Surgery, Gynecology and Obstetrics* 18 (1914): 491-96.
Codman, Ernest Amory. *The Shoulder: Rupture of the Supraspinatus Tendon and Other Lesions in or about the Subacromial Bursa*. Boston: Thomas Todd Company, 1934.
Codman, Ernest Amory. *A Study in Hospital Efficiency: As Demonstrated by the Case Report of the First Five Years of a Private Hospital*. Boston: Thomas Todd Co., 1918.
Cogdell, Christine. *Eugenic Design: Streamlining America in the 1930s*. Philadelphia: University of Pennsylvania Press, 2010.
Cohen, Lizabeth. *Making a New Deal: Industrial Workers in Chicago, 1919-1939*. Cambridge: Cambridge University Press, 1990.

Committee on the Cost of Medical Care. *Medical Care for the American People. The Final Report of the Committee on the Costs of Medical Care, Adopted October 31, 1932.* Chicago: University of Chicago Press, 1932.
"Community Health Meeting Features 2–Day Convention of College of Surgeons." *Brooklyn Daily Eagle*, January 13, 1928.
"Conference on the Standardization of Hospital Practice by Mr. Gilbreth with Dr. Pool and Dr. Bancroft of the New York Hospital," March 1, 1915, MSP 8, box 124, folder 13, Frank and Lillian Gilbreth Library of Management Research and Professional Papers, Purdue University Archives and Special Collections, West Lafayette, IN.
Connor, Steve. "Glaxo Chief: Our Drugs Do Not Work on Most Patients," *The Independent*, December 8, 2003.
Cooper, Alexander. "The Henry Ford Hospital in Time of War: US Army General Hospital No. 36." *Modern Hospital* 14, no. 4 (1920): 259–66.
Cooter, Roger. "'Framing' the End of the Social History of Medicine." In *Locating Medical History: The Stories and Their Meanings*, edited by John Harley Warner and Frank Huisman, 309–37. Baltimore: Johns Hopkins University Press, 2004.
Corwin, Sharon. "Picturing Efficiency: Precisionism, Scientific Management, and the Effacement of Labor." *Representations* 84, no. 1 (2003): 1139–65.
Cowan, Ruth Schwartz. *More Work for Mother: The Ironies of Household Technologies from the Open Hearth to the Microwave.* New York: Basic Books, 1983.
Crenner, Christopher. "Organizational Reform and Professional Dissent in the Careers of Richard Cabot and Ernest Amory Codman, 1900–1920." *Journal of the History of Medicine and Allied Sciences* 56, no. 3 (2001): 211–37.
Crowther, Samuel. "The Real Story of Ford's Hospital." *World's Work* 48 (1924): 540–47.
Cullis, Phillip. "The Limits of Progressivism: Louis Brandeis, Democracy and the Corporation." *Journal of American Studies* 30, no. 3 (1996): 381–404.
Currell, Susan, and Christina Cogdell, eds. *Popular Eugenics: National Efficiency and American Mass Culture in the 1930s.* Athens: Ohio University Press, 2006.
Curtis, Scott. "Images of Efficiency: The Films of Frank B. Gilbreth: Industrial Film and the Productivity of Media." In *Films That Work: Industrial Film and the Productivity of Media*, edited by Vinzenz Hediger and Patrick Vonderau, 85–99. Amsterdam: Amsterdam University Press, 2009.
"Darrow Will Defend Sweet." *Detroit Free Press*, October 16, 1925.
Davis, Loyal. *Fellowship of Surgeons: A History of the American College of Surgeons.* Chicago: American College of Surgeons, [1960] 1996.
Davis, Michael. *America Organizes Medicine.* New York: Harper & Brothers, 1941.
Davis, Michael. "Dispensary and Outpatient Work: How to Make a Dispensary Efficient." *Modern Hospital* 6, no. 4 (1916): 293–94.
Davis, Michael. "Group Medicine." *American Journal of Public Health* 9 (1919): 358–63.
Davis, Michael M. "Problems of Health Service for Negroes." *Journal of Negro Education* 6, no. 3 (1937): 438–49.
"Deformed Boy and Girl Aid Science and Selves." *Oakland Tribune*, October 29, 1935.
DeLee, Joseph. "Before the Baby Comes." *The Delineator*, October 1926, 35, 84.
DeLee, Joseph B. "The Chicago Lying-in Hospital and Dispensary." *Modern Hospital* 4, no. 6 (1915): 383–92.

DeLee, Joseph B. "The Motion Picture in Obstetric Teaching," ca. 1928, box 49, folder 3, Papers of Joseph B. DeLee, Manuscript and Motion Pictures, Northwestern Memorial Hospital Archive, Chicago, IL.

DeLee, Joseph B. "The Prophylactic Forceps Operation." *American Journal of Obstetrics and Gynecology* 40, no. 1 (1920): 34–44.

DeLee, Joseph B., dir. *Science and Art of Obstetrics: Laparotrachalotomy or Low Cervical Section*, 1936, Papers of Joseph B. DeLee, Manuscript and Motion Pictures, Northwestern Memorial Hospital Archive, Chicago, IL.

DeLee, Joseph B. "Sound Motion Pictures in Obstetrics." *Journal of the Biological Photographic Association* 2, no. 2 (1933–34): 60–68.

Derickson, Alan. "Physiological Science and Scientific Management in the Progressive Era: Frederic S. Lee and the Committee on Industrial Fatigue." *Business History Review* 68, no. 4 (1994): 483–514.

Dickinson, Robert L. "Hospital Efficiency from the Standpoint of the Hospital Surgeon." *Boston Medical and Surgical Journal* 172, no. 21 (1915): 775–78.

Dickinson, Robert L. "Standardization of Surgery." *Journal of the American Medical Association* 63, no. 9 (1914): 763–65.

Dickinson, Robert L., and Lura Beam. *The Single Woman: A Medical Study in Sex Education*. Baltimore: Williams & Wilkins, 1934.

Dickinson, Robert L., and Lura Beam. *A Thousand Marriages: A Medical Study of Sex Adjustment*. Baltimore: Williams & Wilkins, 1931.

Dick-Read, Grantly. *Childbirth without Fear: The Principles and Practices of Natural Childbirth*. London: William Heinemann, [1942] 1958.

Dick-Read, Grantly. *Motherhood in the Post-War World*. London: William Heinemann, 1944.

Dick-Read, Grantly. *Natural Childbirth*. London: Heinemann, 1933.

"Distinguished Surgeons Gather in Health Rally at Tucson High School." *Arizona Daily Star*, February 2, 1926.

"Doctors Denounced." *New York Times*, January 21, 1911.

Donabedian, Avedis. "The End Results of Health Care: Ernest Codman's Contribution to Quality Assessment and Beyond." *Milbank Quarterly* 67 (1989): 233–56.

"Dr. Brady's Health Talks: Some Surgeons Are Poor Waiters." *Nebraska State Journal*, May 14, 1933.

"Dr. Mayo Hails New Drive on Germs." *Pittsburgh Sun-Telegraph*, October 12, 1933.

Dublin, Louis. *Health and Wealth: A Survey of the Economics of World Health*. New York: Harper & Brothers, 1928.

Du Bois, W. E. B. *The Philadelphia Negro: A Social Study*. Philadelphia: University of Pennsylvania Press, [1898] 1996.

Du Bois, W. E. B. "The Talented Tenth." In *The Negro Problem*, edited by Booker T. Washington, 31–76. New York: J. Pott, 1903.

Duden, Barbara. *The Woman Beneath the Skin: A Doctor's Patients in Eighteenth-Century Germany*. Translated by Thomas Dunlap. Cambridge, MA: Harvard University Press, 1998.

Duffield, Warren L. "The Hospital Surgeon: His Economics and the Standardization of His Work." *New York State Journal of Medicine* 17, no. 8 (1917): 379–82.

Duffy, Thomas. "The Flexner Report—100 Years Later." *Yale Journal of Biology and Medicine* 84 (2011): 279-86.
Dunott, Daniel. "Report of Recommendations of the American Railway Association in Connection with Hospital Standardization." *Bulletin of the American College of Surgeons* 6, no. 2 (1922): 13-14.
Du Puy, William Atherton. "Henry Ford, of Dearborn, and Some of His Pet Plans." *The Dispatch*, February 16, 1922.
Durkin, Katelyn. "The (Re)production Craze: Taylorism and Regress in Edith Wharton's *Twilight Sleep*." *Edith Wharton Review* 29, no. 2 (2013): 51-74.
Dye, Nancy Schrom. "History of Childbirth in America." *Signs* 6, no. 1 (1980): 97-108.
"Editorial: The Annual Secretarial Conference at Chicago." *New York State Journal of Medicine* 25, no. 23 (1925): 1074-75.
"Editorial: The College of Surgeons." *New York Medical Journal* 98, no. 2 (1913): 91-92.
Esch, Elizabeth. *The Color Line and the Assembly Line: Managing Race in the Ford Empire*. Oakland: University of California Press, 2018.
"Exclusiveism and Specialism in Medical Organizations." *Journal of the American Medical Association* 7, no. 4 (1886): 14-15.
Executive Committee Meeting Minutes, October 9, 1933. RG4/SG04/S02, Minutes of the Board of Regents, the Board of Governors, the Fellows, and Committees. Archives of the American College of Surgeons, Chicago, IL.
Executive Committee Meeting Minutes, June 10, 1934. RG4/SG04/S02, Minutes of the Board of Regents, the Board of Governors, the Fellows, and Committees. Archives of the American College of Surgeons, Chicago, IL.
Field, Alexander J. *A Great Leap Forward: 1930s Depression and Economic Growth*. New Haven, CT: Yale University Press, 2011.
Fields, Anne, and Tschera Harkness Connell. "Classification and the Definition of a Discipline: The Dewey Decimal Classification and Home Economics." *Libraries and Culture* 39, no. 3 (2004): 245-59.
Filene, Edward. "The Minimum Wage and Efficiency." *American Economic Review* 13 (1923): 411-15.
Finney, J. M. T. "The Standardization of the Surgeon." *Journal of the American Medical Association* 63, no. 17 (1914): 1433-37.
Fishbein, Morris. "The Committee on the Costs of Medical Care." *Journal of the American Medical Association* 99, no. 23 (1932): 1950-52.
Fishbein, Morris. "The Report of the Committee on the Costs of Medical Care." *Journal of the American Medical Association* 99, no. 24 (1932): 2034-35.
Fletcher, Horace. *Fletcherism: What It Is or How I Became Young at Sixty*. New York: Frederick Stokes, 1913.
Flexner, Abraham. "Adjusting the College to American Life." *Science*, March 5, 1909, 361-71.
Flexner, Abraham. *The American College: A Criticism*. New York: Century Company, 1908.
Flexner, Abraham. "Aristocratic and Democratic Education." *Atlantic Monthly* (September 1911): 386-95.
Flexner, Abraham. "The German Side of Medical Education." *Atlantic Monthly* (November 1913): 654-62.

Flexner, Abraham. *I Remember: The Autobiography of Abraham Flexner*. New York: Simon & Schuster, 1940.
Flexner, Abraham. *Medical Education*. New York: Macmillan, 1925.
Flexner, Abraham. "Medical Education in America." *Atlantic Monthly* (June 1910): 797–804.
Flexner, Abraham. *Medical Education in the United States and Canada: A Report to the Carnegie Foundation for the Advancement of Teaching*. New York: Carnegie Foundation, 1910.
Flexner, Abraham. *A Modern College and a Modern School*. New York: Doubleday, 1923.
Flexner, Abraham, to Henry Pritchett, April 27, 1921, General Education Board (GEB) file 418, Abraham Flexner Papers, Library of Congress, Washington, DC.
Foote, Christopher, Warren Whatley, and Gavin Wright, "Arbitraging a Discriminatory Labor Market: Black Workers at the Ford Motor Company, 1918–1947." *Journal of Labor Economics* 21, no. 3 (2003): 493–532.
Forbes, Edgar Allan. "Too Many Medical Schools." *World's Work* 20 (1910): 13164–71.
Ford, Henry, and Samuel Crowther. "Greatest Goal in Disease Prevention, Asserts Ford." *San Francisco Chronicle*, May 29, 1926.
Ford, Henry, and Samuel Crowther. "My Life and Work: Chapter IV." *McClure's Magazine* 54, no. 4 (1922): 26–36.
Ford, Henry, and Samuel Crowther. *Today and Tomorrow*. London: William Heinemann, 1926.
"Ford Hospital Aims to Put Health Service on Economic Business Basis." *San Francisco Examiner*, May 28, 1926.
"Ford Hospital Head Quits Surgeons' Body." *Detroit Free Press*, April 30, 1924.
"Ford Hospital in Detroit." *Lincoln State Journal*, March 5, 1926.
"Ford Profit-Sharing Plan Is Explained." *Sacramento Bee*, August 1, 1914.
"Formal Opening of Clinic Attracts Hundreds of People." *Rochester Post and Record*, March 7, 1914.
Foster, William Trufant. "Dollars, Doctors, and Disease." *Atlantic Monthly* (January 1933): 89–96.
Foster, Willian Trufant. "Planning in a Free Country: Managed Money and Unmanaged Men." *Annals of the American Academy of Political and Social Science* 162 (1932): 49–57.
Foster, William Trufant, and Waddill Catchings. *Business without a Buyer*. New York: Houghton Mifflin, 1928.
Fox, Daniel. "Abraham Flexner's Unpublished Report: Foundations and Medical Education." *Bulletin of the History of Medicine*, 54, no. 4 (1980): 475–96.
Fox, Daniel. *Health Policies, Health Politics*. Princeton, NJ: Princeton University Press, 1986.
Frankford, David M. "The Remarkable Staying Power of 'Death Panels.'" *Journal of Health Politics and Policy Law* 40, no. 5 (2015): 1087–101.
"Free Clinics Damage to Doctors Says Fr. Brennan." *Boston Globe*, October 18, 1934.
Freidson, Eliot. *Profession of Medicine. A Study of the Sociology of Applied Knowledge*. Chicago: University of Chicago Press, 1970.
Gainty, Caitjan. "The Autobiographical *Shoulder* of Ernest Amory Codman: Crafting Medical Meaning in the Twentieth Century." *Bulletin of the History of Medicine* 90, no. 3 (2016): 394–423.

Gainty, Caitjan. "A Bit of Hollywood in the Operating Room." *Medicine on Screen: Films and Essays from* NLM. Accessed February 1, 2024. https://medicineonscreen.nlm.nih.gov/2019/07/16/a-bit-of-hollywood-in-the-operating-room/#_edn1.

Gainty, Caitjan. "'Going after the High-Brows': Frank Gilbreth and the Surgical Subject, 1912-1917." *Representations* 118, no. 1 (2012): 1-27.

Gainty, Caitjan. "'Items for Criticism (Not in Sequence)': Joseph DeLee, Pare Lorentz and *The Fight for Life* (1940)." *British Journal for the History of Science* 50, no. 3 (2017): 429-49.

Gainty, Caitjan. "Why Wait?" *Modern American History* 2, no. 2 (2019): 249-55.

Gamble, Vanessa Northington. *Making a Place for Ourselves: The Black Hospital Movement, 1920-1945*. London: Oxford University Press, 1995.

Gamble, Vanessa Northington. "The Negro Hospital Renaissance: The Black Hospital Movement, 1920-1945." In *The American General Hospital: Communities and Social Contexts*, edited by Diana Elizabeth Long and Janet Golden, 82-105. Ithaca, NY: Cornell University Press, 1989.

Garceau, Oliver. "Organized Medicine Enforces Its 'Party Line.'" *The Public Opinion Quarterly* 4, no. 3 (1940): 408-19.

Garceau, Oliver. *Political Life of the American Medical Association*. Cambridge, MA: Harvard University Press, 1941.

Getzen, Thomas. "A 'Brand Name Firm' Theory of Medical Group Practice." *Journal of Industrial Economics* 33, no. 2 (1984): 199-215.

Gilbert, Eleanor. "A Woman Interviews Henry Ford." *Printer's Ink* 121 (1922): 127-37.

Gilbreth, Frank. "Hospital Efficiency from the Standpoint of the Efficiency Expert." *Boston Medical and Surgical Journal* 172 (1915): 774-75.

Gilbreth, Frank. "Motion Study in Surgery." *Canadian Journal of Medicine and Surgery* 40 (1916): 22-31.

Gilbreth, Frank. "Scientific Management in the Hospital." *Modern Hospital* 3 (1914): 321-24.

Gilbreth, Frank. "Untitled Speech," Taylor Society, December 31, 1916, MSP 8, box 96, folder 11, Frank and Lillian Gilbreth Library of Management Research and Professional Papers, Purdue University Archives and Special Collections, West Lafayette, IN.

Gilbreth, Frank, and Lillian Gilbreth. *Fatigue Study: The Elimination of Humanity's Greatest Unnecessary Waste*. New York: Sturgis and Walton, 1916.

Gilbreth, Frank, and Lillian Gilbreth. "Hospital Study." Unpublished manuscript, n.d., ca 1915, MSP 8, box 125, folder 1, Frank and Lillian Gilbreth Library of Management Research and Professional Papers, Purdue University Archives and Special Collections, West Lafayette, IN.

Goldwater, S. S. "Dispensaries: A Growing Factor in Curative and Preventive Medicine." *Boston Medical and Surgical Journal* 172, no. 17 (1915): 613-17.

Goldwater, S. S., to Ernest Amory Codman, December 10, 1913, B MS c60, box 2, folder 26, Ernest Amory Codman Papers, 1849-1981, Francis A. Countway Library of Medicine, Boston, MA.

"Gospel of Cleanliness and Thrift Preached to Army of Ford Employees." *Detroit Evening Times*, April 18, 1914.

"Graft at the Bottom." *Los Angeles Times*, Dec 24, 1913.

Graham, Laurel. "Domesticating Efficiency: Lillian Gilbreth's Scientific Management of Homemakers, 1924-1930." *Signs* 24, no. 3 (1999): 633-75.

Gramsci, Antonio. "From 'Americanism and Fordism.'" In *Social Theory: A Reader*, edited by Jonathan Joseph, 95-100. Edinburgh: Edinburgh University Press, 2005.

Granitz, Elizabeth, and Benjamin Klein. "Monopolization by 'Raising Rivals' Costs': The Standard Oil Case." *Journal of Law and Economics* 39, no. 1 (1996): 1-47.

Green, H. M. "Annual Address of the President of the National Medical Association." *Journal of the National Medical Association* 14, no. 4 (1922): 215-20.

Green, H. M. "A Brief Study of the Hospital Situation among Negroes." *Journal of the National Medical Association* 22, no. 3 (1930): 112-14.

Green, H. M. "President's Address." *Journal of the National Medical Association* 19, no. 1 (1927): 16-21.

Greenleaf, William. *From These Beginnings: The Early Philanthropies of Henry and Edsel Ford, 1911-1936*. Detroit: Wayne State University Press, 1964.

Gressley, Gene, ed. *Voltaire and the Cowboy: The Letters of Thurman Arnold*. Boulder: Colorado Associated University Press, 1977.

Grimm, Eleanor K. "Notebooks," RG5/SG7/S2, reels 32-34. Archives of the American College of Surgeons, Chicago, IL.

Haber, Samuel. *Efficiency and Uplift: Scientific Management in the Progressive Era, 1890-1920*. Chicago: University of Chicago Press, 1973.

Haire, Doris. "The Cultural Warping of Childbirth: A Special Report." Hillsdale, NJ: International Childbirth Education Association, 1972.

Hannsgen, Greg, and Dimitri Papadimitriou. "Did the New Deal Prolong or Worsen the Great Depression?" *Challenge* 53, no. 1 (2010): 63-86.

Harris, Michael R. *Five Counterrevolutionaries in Higher Education: Irving Babbitt, Albert Jay Nock, Abraham Flexner, Robert Maynard Hutchins, Alexander Meiklejohn*. Corvallis: Oregon State University Press, 1970.

Harris, Rowland H., to Abraham Flexner, April 24, 1910. Professional Education file B 95, Abraham Flexner Papers, 1865-1989, Library of Congress, Washington, DC.

Hartley, Earl. "The Forgotten History of Defunct Black Medical Schools in the 19th and 20th Centuries and the Impact of the Flexner Report." *Journal of the National Medical Association* 98, no. 9 (2006): 1425-29.

Hawthorne, Daniel. "Better Hospitals for Everybody." *World's Work* 40, no. 2 (1920): 202-8.

Hays, Samuel. *Conservation and the Gospel of Efficiency: The Progressive Conservation Movement*. Pittsburgh: University of Pittsburgh Press, 1959.

Hays, Will. "Medical Motion Pictures." Meeting of the Board of Governors and Fellows, October 15, 1931, 13-17. Archives of the American College of Surgeons, Chicago, IL.

"Health Systems Decried." *New York Times*, April 1, 1949, 28.

"Henry Ford's Latest Action Both Unfair and Unwise." *Sacramento Bee*, June 16, 1914.

"Henry Ford to Spend Millions to Fight Cancer." *The News-Herald*, June 26, 1914.

"Here's Text of Board's Report on Hospital." *Tampa Tribune*, October 31, 1938.

"Hints for Hospital Superintendents." *Modern Hospital* 4, no. 1 (1915): 72.

Hirshberg, Leonard Keene. "Cities Should Maintain Free Diagnostic Clinics." *Indianapolis Star*, October 24, 1918.

Hirshfield, Daniel. *The Lost Reform: The Campaign for Compulsory Health Insurance in the United States from 1932 to 1943.* Cambridge, MA: Harvard University Press, 1970.
"Home-Made Hospital Appliances." *Modern Hospital* 3, no. 1 (July 1914): 42.
"Home-Made Hospital Appliances." *Modern Hospital* 3, no. 2 (August 1914): 131-32.
"Home-Made Hospital Appliances." *Modern Hospital* 3, no. 4 (October 1914): 267.
"Home-Made Hospital Appliances." *Modern Hospital* 3, no. 5 (November 1914): 330-37.
"Home-Made Hospital Appliances: Devices Improvised in Institutions to Lighten the Work or to Make It More Efficient." *Modern Hospital* 3, no. 1 (July 1914): 51-52.
Hooker, Clarence. "Ford's Sociology Department and the Americanization Campaign and the Manufacture of Popular Culture among Assembly Line Workers c. 1910-1917." *Journal of American Culture* 20, no. 1 (1997): 47-53.
Hornsby, John. "How a Great Clinic Works." *Modern Hospital* 10, no. 5 (1918): 333-35.
"Hospital Betterment in California." *California State Journal of Medicine* 19, no. 7 (1921): 261.
Hospital Conference of the American College of Surgeons, October 22-23, 1923. American College of Surgeons Archives, Chicago, IL.
"Hospital Cost Standardized: Angelus Institution Adopts Revolutionary Plan." *Los Angeles Times*, February 20, 1928.
"Hospital Standardization Conference." *Bulletin of the American College of Surgeons* 4, no. 3 (1920): 3-9.
"Hospitals Big Asset to City." *Great Falls Tribune*, September 17, 1923.
Hounshell, David. *From the American System to Mass Production, 1800-1932: The Development of Manufacturing Technology in the United States.* Baltimore: Johns Hopkins University Press, 1984.
Howell, Joel. *Technology in the Hospital: Transforming Patient Care in the Early Twentieth Century.* Baltimore: Johns Hopkins University Press, 1995.
Hoxie, Robert F. "Organized Labor and Industrial Efficiency." *American Review of Reviews* 44 (1911): 482-83.
Hoxie, Robert F. "Why Organized Labor Opposes Scientific Management." *Quarterly Journal of Economics* 13 (1917): 62-85.
Hudson, Robert P. "Abraham Flexner in Perspective: American Medical Education 1865-1910." *Bulletin of the History of Medicine* 46, no. 6 (1972): 545-61.
Hyde, Alan. *Bodies of Law.* Princeton, NJ: Princeton University Press, 1997.
Illich, Ivan. *Limits to Medicine.* New York: Marion Boyars, 1995.
Illich, Ivan. *Medical Nemesis: The Expropriation of Health.* New York: Pantheon Books, [1974] 1977.
Jackson, Algernon Brashear. "Hospitals and Health." *Journal of the National Medical Association* 22, no. 3 (1930): 115-19.
Jackson, Edward. "Letter to the Editor: Doctor and Patient." *Journal of the American Medical Association* 110, no. 17 (1938): 1386-87.
"Joint Commission History Timeline." The Joint Commission. Accessed February 20, 2024. https://www.jointcommission.org/-/media/tjc/documents/tjc-history-timeline-through-2022.pdf.
Jones, Jane Clare. "Idealized and Industrialized Labor: Anatomy of a Feminist Controversy." *Hypatia* 27, no. 1 (2012): 99-117.

Jones, Philip Mills. "The American Royal College of Surgeons—J. B. M." *California State Journal of Medicine* 11, no. 5 (1913): 175–76.

Jones, Philip Mills. "The American Royal Surgical Emporium." *California State Journal of Medicine* 11, no. 6 (1913): 212.

Jones, Philip Mills. "Congress of Surgeons." *California State Journal of Medicine* 11, no. 11 (1913): 473.

Jones, Philip Mills. "The Costume of the College." *California State Journal of Medicine* 12, no. 2 (1914): 47.

Jones, Philip Mills. "Is the Clinical Congress an Unmixed Blessing?" *California State Journal of Medicine* 11, no. 10 (1913): 388.

"Just a Word." *The Independent*, October 26, 1914, 113.

Kaempffert, Waldemar. "Diagnosing the Case of Organized Medicine Today." *New York Times*, May 21, 1939.

Kaempffert, Waldemar. "Speaking of Doctors and How They Take Care of You: A Thorough and Objective Study of Medical Care in America by Michael Davis." *New York Times*, August 17, 1941.

Kanavel, Allen. "The Hospital as an Educational Center." Conference on Hospital Standardization, October, 19–20, 1917. Archives of the American College of Surgeons, Chicago, IL.

Kanigel, Robert. *The One Best Way: Frederick Winslow Taylor and the Enigma of Efficiency.* New York: Penguin-Viking, 1997.

Kellogg, J. H. *The Itinerary of a Breakfast.* New York: Funk and Wagnalls, 1919.

Kellogg, J. H. *The Stomach: Its Disorders and How to Cure Them.* Battle Creek, MI: Modern Medicine Publishing, 1896.

Kelly, J. E. *Scientific Management, Job Redesign and Work Performance.* New York: Academic Press, 1982.

Kenney, John. "The Negro Hospital Renaissance." *Journal of the National Medical Association* 22, no. 3 (1930): 109–12.

Kenney, John. "Why a National Hospital Association?" *Journal of the National Medical Association* 18, no. 3 (1926): 138–39.

Kenney, John A. *The Negro in Medicine.* Tuskegee, AL: Tuskegee Institute Press, 1912.

Kessel, Reuben A. "Price Discrimination in Medicine." *Journal of Law and Economics* 1 (1958): 20–53.

King, Lester. "The Flexner Report of 1910." *Journal of the American Medical Association* 251, no. 8 (1984): 1071–86.

Kisacky, Jeanne. *Rise of the Modern Hospital: An Architectural History of Health and Healing, 1870–1940.* Pittsburgh: University of Pittsburgh Press, 2017.

Kline, Wendy. "Back to Bed: From Hospital to Home Obstetrics in the City of Chicago." *Journal of the History of Medicine and Allied Sciences* 73, no. 1 (2018): 29–51.

Kline, Wendy. *Bodies of Knowledge: Sexuality, Reproduction, and Women's Health in the Second Wave.* Chicago: University of Chicago Press, 2010.

Kline, Wendy. "How to Train an Obstetrician: Lessons from the Chicago Maternity Center." *Process: A Blog for American History*, January 26, 2017. http://www.processhistory.org/kline-train-obstetrician/.

Kraines, Oscar. "Brandeis' Philosophy of Scientific Management." *The Western Political Quarterly* 13, no. 1 (1960): 191–201.
Kyrk, Hazel. *A Theory of Consumption*. Boston: Houghton Mifflin, 1923.
Lalvani, Suren. *Photography, Vision, and the Production of Modern Bodies*. Albany, NY: SUNY Press, 1996.
Lamoreaux, Naomi R. "The Problem of Bigness: From Standard Oil to Google." *Journal of Economic Perspectives* 33, no. 3 (2019): 94–117.
Lampland, Martha, and Susan Leigh Star, eds. *Standards and Their Stories. How Quantifying, Classifying, and Formalizing Practices Shape Everyday Life*. Ithaca, NY: Cornell University Press, 2009.
Laurence, William. "Health Insurance Gets Official Aid." *New York Times*, October 16, 1934.
Laurence, William. "Nation's Doctors Called to Revolt." *New York Times*, April 7, 1938, 1, 24.
Laurence, William. "To Urge Reduction in Hospital Costs." *New York Times*, October 15, 1934.
Leavitt, Judith Walzer. *Brought to Bed: Childbearing in America, 1750–1950*. New York: Oxford University Press, [1987] 2017.
Leavitt, Judith Walzer. "Joseph B. DeLee and the Practice of Preventive Obstetrics." *American Journal of Public Health* 78, no. 10 (1988): 1353–60.
Leavitt, Judith Walzer. "Science Enters the Birthing Room: Obstetrics in America since the Eighteenth Century." *Journal of American History* 70, no. 2 (1983): 281–304.
Leavitt, Judith Walzer. *Typhoid Mary: Captive to the Public's Health*. Boston: Beacon Press, 1996.
Lee, John. "The So-Called Profit Sharing System in the Ford Plant." *Annals of the American Academy of Political and Social Science* 65 (1916): 297–310.
Leven, Maurice, Harold G. Moulton, and Clark Warburton. *America's Capacity to Consume*. Washington, DC: Brookings Institution, 1935.
Lewis, H. Edwin. "Editorial: Weak Medical Schools as Nurseries of Medical Genius." *American Medicine* 17, no. 9 (1911): 447–48.
Lewis, Sinclair. *The Man Who Knew Coolidge*. New York: Harcourt Brace, 1928.
Lichtenstein, Diane. "Domestic Novels of the 1920s: Regulation and Efficiency in *The Home-Maker, Twilight Sleep,* and *Too Much Efficiency*." *American Studies* 52, no. 2 (2013): 65–88.
"Lid Off in Hospital Row." *Tampa Tribune*, October 31, 1938.
Liebes, Herman, to Helen Joseph, April 28, 1963, box 49, folder 2, Papers of Joseph B. DeLee, Manuscript and Motion Pictures, Northwestern Memorial Hospital Archive, Chicago, IL.
"Lincoln Hears Doctors." *Lincoln State Journal*, February 7, 1922.
Lindstrom, Richard. "'They All Believe They Are Undiscovered Mary Pickfords': Workers, Photography, and Scientific Management." *Technology and Culture* 41, no. 4 (2000): 725–51.
Link, Stefan. *Forging Global Fordism: Nazi Germany, Soviet Russia, and the Contest over the Industrial Order*. Princeton, NJ: Princeton University Press, 2020.
"Local Hospital Given Approval." *Indiana Gazette*, October 27, 1925.
Loizides, Gergios, and Subhash Sonnad. "Fordist Applied Research in the Era of the Five-Dollar Day." *Sociological Practice* 6, no. 2 (2004): 1–25.

Long, Durward. "An Immigrant Co-Operative Medicine Program in the South, 1887-1963." *Journal of Southern History* 31, no. 4 (1965): 417-34.

Ludmerer, Kenneth. *Learning to Heal*. Baltimore: Johns Hopkins University Press, 1985.

Lupton, Ellen H., and Abbott Miller. *The Bathroom, the Kitchen and the Aesthetics of Waste: A Process of Elimination*. Cambridge, MA: MIT List Visual Arts Center, 1992.

Lydston, G. Frank. "Medicine as a Business Proposition." *Journal of the American Medical Association* 34, no. 22 (1900): 1400-1404.

Lynn, Harrison. *The Crime of the Century: An Exposure of the Inner Methods of the American Medical Association*. Battle Creek, MI: Truth Teller Publishing, 1915.

Magill, Thomas. "The Immunologist and the Evil Spirits." *Journal of Immunology* 74 (1955): 1-8.

Mandell, Mike. *Making Good Time: Scientific Management, the Gilbreths' Photography and Motion Futurism*. Santa Cruz, CA: Mike Mandell, 1989.

Markowitz, Gerald E., and David Karl Rosner. "Doctors in Crisis: A Study of the Use of Medical Education Reform to Establish Modern Professional Elitism in Medicine." *American Quarterly* 25, no. 1 (1973): 83-107.

Martin, D. D. "Henry Ford Hospital in Time of Peace." *Modern Hospital* 14, no. 4 (1920): 266-70.

Martin, Franklin. "The American College of Surgeons and Better Hospitals." Hospital Conference, October 22-23, 1923. Archives of the American College of Surgeons, Chicago, IL.

Mavity, Nancy Barr. "Surgeons at S. F. Congress to Banish Fear of Knife at Mass Meeting Tonight." *Oakland Tribune*, October 30, 1935.

Mayers, Lewis, and Leonard V. Harrison. *The Distribution of Physicians in the United States*. New York: General Education Board, 1924.

Mayo, Charles H. "Nature, Value and Necessity of Teamwork in a Hospital." *Modern Hospital* 7, no. 1 (1916): 1-3.

"Mayo Clinic Building Is Formally Opened, The." *Rochester Daily Bulletin*, March 7, 1914.

"Mayor Plans to Have City Take Over and Operate Detroit General Hospital." *Detroit Times*, May 21, 1914.

McCormick, Edward J. "Dr. Malcom T. MacEachern Retires as Head of Approval Program." *Hospital Management* 70, no. 5 (1950): 23-24.

McEvoy, J. P. "Our Streamlined Baby." *Reader's Digest* (May 1938): 15-18.

McFeeley, Otto. "Ford Consumptives Cured at Work: System Has Yet to Lose Patient." *Detroit Times*, January 25, 1914.

McFeeley, Otto. "Will Spend Millions in New Hospital in Finding Ways to Prevent Scourge." *Detroit Times*, June 26, 1914.

McKeown, Thomas. *The Role of Medicine: Dream, Mirage or Nemesis*. London: Nuffield Trust, 1976.

McKeown, Thomas, and R. G. Record. "Medical Evidence Related to English Population Changes in the Eighteenth Century." *Population Studies* 9, no. 2 (1955): 119-41.

McKeown, Thomas, and R. G. Record. "Reasons for the Decline of Mortality in England and Wales during the Nineteenth Century." *Population Studies* 16, no. 2 (1962): 94-122.

"Medical Leaders Organize to Fight Destructive Propaganda." *St. Cloud Times*, December 30, 1939.

"Medical Motion Pictures." Meeting of Board of Governors and Fellows, October 15, 1931, 13-17. Archives of the American College of Surgeons, Chicago, IL.

"Medical Schools of the United States." *Journal of the American Medical Association* 51, no. 7 (1908): 599-602.

"Medical Science Beating Disease, Statistics Show." *Oakland Tribune*, October 29, 1935.

"Medical Trust Makes Fight." *Indianapolis Star*, July 12, 1912.

Meiksins, Peter F. "Scientific Management and Class Relations: A Dissenting View." *Theory and Society* 13, no. 2 (1984): 177-209.

"Men and Things." *American Medicine* 16, no. 10 (1910): 504-5.

Merkle, Judith A. *Management and Ideology: The Legacy of the International Scientific Management Movement*. Berkeley: University of California Press, 1980.

Meyer, Stephen. "Adapting the Immigrant to the Line: Americanization in the Ford Factory, 1914-1921." *Journal of Social History* 14, no. 10 (1980): 67-82.

Michaels, Paula. *Lamaze: An International History*. London: Oxford University Press, 2014.

Miller, Lynn E., and Richard M. Weiss. "Revisiting Black Medical School Extinctions in the Flexner Era." *Journal of the History of Medicine and Allied Sciences* 67, no. 2 (2012): 217-43.

"Minutes of the Third Annual Session of the National Hospital Association." *Journal of the National Medical Association* 17, no. 4 (1925): 229-33.

"Monopoly Move Hailed by G.H.A." *Washington Evening Star*, August 1, 1938.

Montgomery, David. *Workers' Control in America: Studies in the History of Work, Technology and Labor Struggles*. Cambridge: Cambridge University Press, 1979.

"More Care of Health Urged by College of Surgeons Public Meeting Here Monday." *Herald and Review*, June 11, 1927.

Morgen, Sandra. *Into Our Own Hands: The Women's Health Movement in the United States, 1969-1990*. New Brunswick, NJ: Rutgers University Press, 2002.

Mormino, Gary R., and George E. Pozzetta. *The Immigrant World of Ybor City: Italians and Their Latin Neighbors in Tampa, 1885-1985*. Gainesville: University of Florida Press, [1987] 2017.

Moscucci, Ornella. "Holistic Obstetrics: The Origins of 'Natural Childbirth' in Britain." *Postgraduate Medical Journal* 79, no. 929 (2003): 168-73.

Moulinier, Charles. "Hospital Standardization and the Medical and Nursing Professions." Hospital Conference of the American College of Surgeons, October 22-23, 1923, 30-34. Archives of the American College of Surgeons, Chicago, IL.

Moulinier, Charles. "The Standardization Program of the American College of Surgeons." *Bulletin of the American College of Surgeons* 6, no. 22 (1922): 11-12.

"Movies Enter New Field of Science Today." *Los Angeles Evening Express*, October 26, 1926.

"Movies to Help Baseball Players Economize Force." *New York Tribune*, June 15, 1913.

"Moving Sidewalks and Other Luxuries." *Modern Hospital* 6, no. 4 (1916): 273.

"Mr. Bynum on the Currency." *New York Times*, September 23, 1896.

Murphy, Michelle. *Seizing the Means of Reproduction: Entanglements of Feminism, Health, and Technoscience*. Durham, NC: Duke University Press, 2012.

Nadworny, Milton J. *Scientific Management and the Unions, 1900-1932: A Historical Analysis*. Cambridge: Cambridge University Press, 1955.

National Medical Association. "Historical Manifesto." Accessed February 29, 2024. https://www.nmanet.org/page/Mission.

Nelson, Daniel. *Frederick W. Taylor and the Rise of Scientific Management*. Madison: University of Wisconsin Press, 1980.
Nelson, Daniel. "Scientific Management and the Workplace, 1920-1935." In *Masters to Managers, Historical and Comparative Perspectives on American Employers*, edited by Sanford Jacoby, 74-89. New York: Columbia University Press, 1991.
Nelson, Jennifer. *More than Medicine: A History of the Feminist Women's Health Movement*. New York: New York University Press, 2015.
Niebuhr, Reinhold. *The Negro in Detroit, Section 6: Health*. Detroit: Detroit Bureau of Governmental Research, 1926.
Noble, David. *America by Design: Science, Technology and the Rise of Corporate Capitalism*. New York: Alfred A. Knopf, 1982.
Noble, David. *Forces of Production: A Social History of Industrial Automation*. New York: Oxford University Press, 1984.
Nock, Albert Jay. "Efficiency and the High-Brow: Frank Gilbreth's Great Plan to Introduce Time-Study into Surgery." *American Magazine* 75, no. 3 (1913): 48-50.
Notes of the Executive Committee meeting, October 9, 1933, Stevens Hotel, Chicago. Archive of the American College of Surgeons, Chicago, IL.
Nyland, Chris. *Reduced Worktime and the Management of Production*. Cambridge: Cambridge University Press, 1989.
Nyland, Chris. "Scientific Management and Planning." *Capital & Class* 11, no. 3 (1987): 55-83.
Nyland, Chris. "Taylorism, John R. Commons, and the Hoxie Report." *Journal of Economic Issues* 30, no. 4 (1996): 985-1016.
"Objects to Ethics of Ford's Hospital." *New York Times*, April 19, 1924.
O'Brien, Anthony Patrick. "A Behavioral Explanation for Nominal Wage Rigidity during the Great Depression." *Quarterly Journal of Economics* 104, no. 4 (1989): 719-35.
O'Brien, Anthony Patrick, Jason Taylor, and George Selgin, "By Our Bootstraps: Origins and Effects of the High-Wage Doctrine and the Minimum Wage." *Journal of Labor Research* 20, no. 4 (1999): 447-61.
"Officials Believe Hospital's Offer Will Be Accepted." *Detroit Free Press*, May 23, 1914.
Olszynko-Gryn, Jesse. *A Woman's Right to Know: Pregnancy Testing in Twentieth-Century Britain*. Cambridge, MA: MIT Press, 2023.
"Oregon Surgeons to Meet on Friday for Conference." *Oregon Daily Journal*, April 10, 1919.
Orgeron, Devin, Marsha Orgeron, and Dan Streible. *Learning with the Lights Off: Educational Film in the United States*. New York: Oxford University Press, 2012.
Orr, Douglas. "Review: *American Medicine Mobilizes*." *Annals of the American Academy of Political and Social Science* 205, no. 1 (1939): 145-46.
Ostherr, Kirsten. "Medical Education through Film: Animating Anatomy at the American College of Surgeons and Eastman Kodak." In *Learning with the Lights Off: Educational Film in the United States*, edited by Devin Orgeron, Marsha Orgeron and Dan Streible, 168-92. New York: Oxford University Press, 2012.
Ostherr, Kirsten. *Medical Visions: Producing the Patient through Film, Television, and Imaging Technologies*. New York: Oxford University Press, 2013.
"Our Hospitals Work for Human Salvage." *The Daily News*, October 13, 1930.
"Oversupply of Medical Graduates." *Journal of the American Medical Association* 37 (1901): 270.

Painter, Patricia Scollard. *Henry Ford Hospital, the First 75 Years*. Detroit: Henry Ford Health System, 1997.
"Patients Watched after Discharge." *Montreal Gazette*, October 20, 1926.
Peterkin, G. Shearman. "Ethical Economics." *California Eclectic Medical Journal* 40 (1919): 127–31.
"Physician: The Plight of the Family Doctor, A." *New York Times*, January 28, 1923.
"Physicians to Give Series of Talks." *Berkshire Eagle*, October 9, 1933.
Pickstone, John. "Medicine, Society and the State." In *The Cambridge Illustrated History of Medicine*, edited by Roy Porter, 304–41. Cambridge: University of Cambridge Press, 1996.
Pietrykowski, Bruce. "Fordism at Ford: Spatial Decentralization and Labor Segmentation at the Ford Motor Company, 1920–1950." *Economic Geography* 71, no. 4 (1995): 383–401.
Plante, Lauren A. "Mommy, What Did You Do in the Industrial Revolution? Meditations on the Rising Cesarean Rate." *International Journal of Feminist Approaches to Bioethics* 2, no. 1 (2009): 140–47.
"Plummer Building." Mayo Clinic Historical Unit, W. Bruce Fye Center for the History of Medicine, Mayo Clinic, Rochester, MN.
Pomeroy, Ross. "1910: The Year American Medicine Changed Forever." *Real Clear Science*, November 8, 2018. https://www.realclearscience.com/blog/2018/11/08/1910_the_year _american_medicine_changed_forever.html.
Pool, Eugene, and Robert Bancroft. "Systematization of a Surgical Service." *Journal of the American Medical Association* 69, no. 9 (1917): 1599–1603.
Pooley, Jefferson. "James Rorty's Voice: Introduction to the Mediastudies.press Edition." In *Our Master's Voice: Advertising*, by James Rorty and Jefferson Pooley, xiv–xxxi. Mediastudies.press, 2020. Project MUSE, https://muse.jhu.edu/book/80832.
Posner, Miriam. "Communicating Disease: Tuberculosis, Narrative, and Social Order in Thomas Edison's Red Cross Seal Films." In *Learning with the Lights Off: Educational Film in the United States*, edited by Devin Orgeron, Marsha Orgeron, and Dan Streible, 90–106. New York: Oxford University Press, 2012.
Pritchett, Henry. "Should the Carnegie Foundation Be Suppressed?" *North American Review* 201, no. 713 (1915): 554–66.
Pritchett, Henry. "Weak Medical Schools as Nurseries of Medical Genius." *Journal of the American Medical Association* 56, no. 8 (1911): 589–91.
Pritchett, Henry, and R. A. Franks. *Fifth Annual Report of the President and Treasurer*. New York: Carnegie Foundation for the Advancement of Teaching, 1910.
"Program of Activity." *Bulletin of the American College of Surgeons* 1, no. 1 (1916): 11–12.
Program of the Community Health Meeting, Wednesday, October 11, 1933. Archives of the American College of Surgeons, Chicago, IL.
"Public Service Aim of Doctors' Society." *Salt Lake City Tribune*, November 23, 1920.
"Public Support Urged to Save Voluntary Hospitals." *Oakland Tribune*, October 28, 1935.
Purinton, Edward. "Efficiency Question Box." *The Independent*, December 21, 1914, 480.
Purinton, Edward. *Efficient Living*. New York: Robert M. McBride, 1915.
Purinton, Edward. *Personal Efficiency in Business*. New York: Sir Isaac Pitman and Sons, Ltd., 1919.

Rabinbach, Anson. *The Human Motor: Energy, Fatigue and the Origins of Modernity*. Berkeley: University of California Press, 1992.

Raub, Benjamin D. "The Anti-Trust Prosecution against the American Medical Association." *Law and Contemporary Problems* 6, no. 4 (1939): 595–605.

Rayack, Elton. *Professional Power and American Medicine: The Economics of the American Medical Association*. Cleveland: World Publishing Company, 1967.

Reed, C. H. "Why Is the Profession Poor in Purse? And How to Remedy It." *Journal of the American Medical Association* 32 (1899): 975.

Reminiscences of Dr. F. Janney Smith, Owen W. Bombard Interviews Series, 1951–1961, Accession 65, digitized transcript, Benson Ford Research Center, The Henry Ford, Dearborn, MI. Accessed March 7, 2024. https://cdm15889.contentdm.oclc.org/digital/collection/p15889coll2/id/15959/rec/7.

Reminiscences of William J. Cameron, Accession 65, box 11, folders 3-4, Owen W. Bombard Interviews Series, Benson Ford Research Center, The Henry Ford, Dearborn, MI.

Reverby, Susan. "Stealing the Golden Eggs: Ernest Amory Codman and the Science and Management of Medicine." *Bulletin of the History of Medicine* 55, no. 2 (1981): 156–71.

Reverby, Susan, and David Rosner. "Beyond 'the Great Doctors.'" In *Health Care in America: Essays in Social Medicine*, edited by Susan Reverby and David Rosner, 3–16. Philadelphia: Temple University Press, 1979.

"Review: American Medicine Mobilizes." *Journal of Educational Sociology* 13, no. 8 (1940): 507.

Richardson, Anna Steese. "'Better Babies,' The Nation's New Slogan." *Los Angeles Times*, May 4, 1913.

Rodengen, Jeffrey L. *Henry Ford Health System: A 100 Year Legacy*. Fort Lauderdale: Write Stuff Enterprises, 2014.

Rogers, Naomi. "Germs with Legs: Flies, Disease, and the New Public Health." *Bulletin of the History of Medicine* 63, no. 4 (1989): 599–617.

Rorty, James. *American Medicine Mobilizes*. New York: W. W. Norton, 1939.

Rorty, James. *Our Master's Voice: Advertising*. New York: John Day Company, 1934.

Rose, Nikolas. "Beyond Medicalisation." *The Lancet* 369 (2007): 700–702.

Rosen, George. "Contract or Lodge Practice and Its Influence on Medical Attitudes to Health Insurance." *American Journal of Public Health* 67 (1977): 374–78.

Rosenberg, Charles. *The Care of Strangers: The Rise of America's Hospital System*. New York: Basic Books, 1987.

Rosenberg, Charles E. "The Tyranny of Diagnosis: Specific Entities and Individual Experience." *Milbank Quarterly* 80, no. 2 (2002): 237–60.

Rutecki, Gregory. "Clinical Science after Flexner's 1910 Report on Medical Education: A Research Ethos Inhabited by Racial Prejudice, Colonial Attitudes and Eugenic Theory." *Ethics and Medicine* 36, no. 1 (2020): 51–62.

Rutkow, Ira. *Seeking the Cure: A History of Medicine in America*. New York: Scribner, 2010.

Savitt, Todd. "Abraham Flexner and the Black Medical Schools." *Journal of the National Medical Association* 98, no. 9 (2006): 1415–24.

Savitt, Todd. "Entering a White Profession: Black Physicians in the New South, 1880-1920." *Bulletin of the History of Medicine* 61, no. 4 (1987): 507–40.

Savitt, Todd. *Race and Medicine in Nineteenth- and Early-Twentieth-Century America*. Kent, OH: Kent State University Press, 2007.

Schachter, H. L. "Democracy, Scientific Management and Urban Reform: The Case of the Bureau of Municipal Research and the 1912 New York City Inquiry." *Journal of Management History* 1 (1995): 52-64.

Schlich, Thomas. *Surgery, Science and Industry: A Revolution in Fracture Care, 1950s-1990s. Science, Technology and Medicine in Modern History.* London: Palgrave, 2002.

Schlich, Thomas. "Trauma Surgery and Traffic Policy in Germany in the 1930s: A Case Study in the Coevolution of Modern Surgery and Society." *Bulletin of the History of Medicine* 80, no. 1 (2006): 73-94.

Schulz, Stanley. "The Morality of Politics: The Muckrakers' Vision of Democracy." *Journal of American History* 52, no. 3 (1965): 527-47.

"Secretary" to Abraham Flexner, March 9, 1914, Professional Education file B 95, Abraham Flexner Papers, Library of Congress, Washington, DC.

Shadid, Michael. *A Doctor for the People: The Autobiography of the Founder of America's First Co-operative Hospital.* New York: Vanguard Press, 1939.

Shadid, Michael. *Doctors of Today and Tomorrow.* New York: Cooperative League of America, 1949.

Shortliffe, Edward. "The Adolescence of AI in Medicine: Will the Field Come of Age in the 1990s?" *Artificial Intelligence and Medicine* 5, no. 2 (1993): 93-106.

Shryock, Richard. "Freedom and Interference in Medicine." *Annals of the American Academy of Political and Social Science* 200 (1938): 32-59.

Shumard, E. C. "Correspondence: Foresight of Henry Ford." *Scientific American* 113, no. 26 (1915): 557.

Sigerist, Henry. *Medicine and Human Welfare.* New Haven, CT: Yale University Press, 1941.

Slobe, Frederick. "The Hospital Survey of the College in 1921." *Bulletin of the American College of Surgeons* 6, no. 2 (1922): 5-8.

"Sprinkle Out as Head Man; Bar 9 Doctors from Staff." *Tampa Evening Tribune*, October 31, 1938.

"Standard of Efficiency: Requirements." *Bulletin of the American College of Surgeons* 3, no. 3 (1918): 1.

Starr, Paul. *The Social Transformation of American Medicine.* New York: Basic Books, 1982.

State Executive Committee Meeting, October 24, 1922. Archives of the American College of Surgeons, Chicago, IL.

Steffens, Lincoln. *The Shame of the Cities.* New York: McClure, Philips, [1902] 1904.

Stevens, Rosemary. *American Medicine and the Public Interest.* New Haven, CT: Yale University Press, 1971.

Stevens, Rosemary. *In Sickness and in Wealth: American Hospitals in the Twentieth Century.* New York: Basic Books, 1989.

Strasser, Susan. "Sponsorship and Snake Oil: Medicine Shows and Contemporary Public Culture." In *Public Culture: Diversity, Democracy, and Community in the United States*, edited by Marguerite S. Shaffer, 91-113. Philadelphia: University of Pennsylvania Press, 2008.

Sturdy, Steve, and Roger Cooter. "Science, Scientific Management and the Transformation of Medicine in Britain, 1870-1950." *History of Science* 36, no. 4 (1998): 421-66.

"Surgeons Attack Ford Hospital System; Say Patients Are Overhauled Like Autos." *New York Times*, April 13, 1924.

"Surgeons Here Stack Up with Best—Franklin." *Tucson Citizen*, February 1, 1926.

"Surgeons Make a Hospital Survey." *Battle Creek Enquirer*, October 20, 1924.
"Surgeons Open Sectional Meet in City Today." *Arizona Daily Star*, February 1, 1926.
"Surgeons Perform Miracle of Science." *Oakland Tribune*, April 25, 1931.
"Surgeons Spend Busy Day Here." *Nashville Banner*, March 22, 1921.
Tarbell, Ida. "Fear of Efficiency." *The Independent*, July 7, 1917, 19–21.
Tarbell, Ida. *The History of the Standard Oil Company*. New York: McClure, Philips, 1904.
Tarr, G. Alan. "Laboratories of Democracy?: Brandeis, Federalism and Scientific Management." *Publius* 31, no. 1 (2001): 37–46.
Taylor, Frederick Winslow. *The Principles of Scientific Management*. New York: Harper and Brothers, 1911.
"Ten Are Held for Murder in Race Conflict." *Detroit Free Press*, September 11, 1925.
Tenner, Edward. "The Technological Imperative." *The Wilson Quarterly (1976–)* 19, no. 1 (1995): 26–34.
Thirkield, Wilbur, to Henry Pritchett, February 21, 1910, Professional Education file B 95, Abraham Flexner Papers, Library of Congress, Washington, DC.
Thomas, Samuel. "Holding the Tiger: Mugwump Cartoonists and Tammany Hall in Gilded Age New York." *New York History* 82, no. 2 (2001): 155–82.
Thomas, Vivien. *Partners of the Heart: Vivien Thomas and His Work with Alfred Blalock*. Philadelphia: University of Pennsylvania Press, 1985.
Thorning, Joseph F. "Social Medicine in Cuba. El Centro Asturiano, La Habana." *The Americas* 1, no. 4 (1945): 440–55.
Tichi, Cecelia. *Exposés and Excess: Muckraking in America, 1900/2000*. Philadelphia: University of Pennsylvania Press, 2004.
Timmermans, Stefan, and Marc Berg. *The Gold Standard: The Challenge of Evidence-Based Medicine and Standardization in Health Care*. Philadelphia: Temple University Press, 2003.
Timmermans, Stefan, and Steven Epstein. "A World of Standards but Not a Standard World: Toward a Sociology of Standards and Standardization." *Annual Review of Sociology* 36 (2010): 69–89.
"Today in Tucson," *Arizona Daily Star*, February 1, 1926, 1.
Tomes, Nancy. "Comment: What Historians of Medicine Can Learn from Historians of Capitalism." *Bulletin of the History of Medicine* 94, no. 3 (2020): 374–83.
Tomes, Nancy. "Epidemic Entertainments: Disease and Popular Culture in Early-Twentieth-Century America." *American Literary History* 14, no. 4 (2002): 625–52.
Tomes, Nancy. *The Gospel of Germs: Men, Women and the Microbe in American Life*. Cambridge, MA: Harvard University Press, 1998.
Tomes, Nancy. "Merchants of Health: Medicine and Consumer Culture in the United States, 1900–1940." *Journal of American History* 88, no. 2 (2001): 519–47.
Tomes, Nancy. *Remaking the American Patient: How Madison Avenue and Modern Medicine Turned Patients into Consumers*. Chapel Hill: University of North Carolina Press, 2016.
Tone, Andrea. *Devices and Desires: A History of Contraceptives in America*. New York: Hill & Wang, 2002.
Tone, Andrea. "Medicalizing Reproduction: The Pill and Home Pregnancy Tests." *Journal of Sex Research* 49, no. 4 (2012): 319–27.
Tugwell, Rexford G. *Industry's Coming of Age*. New York: Harcourt, Brace, 1927.
United States v. American Medical Association et al. 28 F. Supp. 752, 755 (D. D. C. 1939).

"US Hospitals for Veterans Are Attacked." *Oakland Tribune*, October 30, 1935.

Valentine, Robert G. "Application of Principles of Organization to Hospital Service: Organization Is Not a Fetish, Not a Mechanical Figure, but a Flexible, Living Thing Which All Forces Are Marshaled for Achievement—The Patient Is the Center and Object of Hospital Service." *Modern Hospital* 6, no. 4 (1916): 262-67.

"Vital Importance Child Welfare Work Urged in Rousing Addresses at Community Health Gathering." *Ottawa Citizen*, November 23, 1923.

"Vital Importance of Early Medical Attention Stressed at Surgeons' Mass Meeting." *The Asheville Citizen*, March 21, 1922.

Vogel, Morris. *The Invention of the Modern Hospital: Boston, 1870-1930*. Chicago: University of Chicago Press, 1980.

Vogel, Morris J., and Charles Rosenberg, eds. *The Therapeutic Revolution: Essays in the Social History of American Medicine*. Philadelphia: University of Pennsylvania Press, 1979.

Von Neupert, Carl. "Dr. Carl von Neupert Discusses American College of Surgeons." *Stevens Point Daily Journal*, March 13, 1930.

Ward, Patricia Spain. "United States versus American Medical Association et al.: The Medical Antitrust Case of 1938-1943." *American Studies* 30, no. 2 (1989): 123-53.

Warner, John Harley. "The Aesthetic Grounding of Modern Medicine." *Bulletin of the History of Medicine* 88, no. 1 (2014): 1-47.

Warner, John Harley. "The History of Science and the Sciences of Medicine." *Osiris* 10 (1995): 164-93.

Warner, John Harley. "Science in Medicine." *Osiris* 1 (1985): 37-58.

Warner, John Harley. *The Therapeutic Perspective: Medical Practice, Knowledge and Identity in America, 1820-1885*. Cambridge, MA: Harvard University Press, 1986.

Washburn, S. S. "Standardized Home-Made Appliances." *Modern Hospital* 3, no. 2 (1914): 131-33.

Washington, Booker T. *Industrial Education for the Negro*. Tuskegee, AL: Tuskegee Institute, 1904.

Washington, Booker T. *The Negro Problem*. New York: James Pott, 1903.

Weiss, Richard M., and Lynn E. Miller. "The Social Transformation of American Medical Education: Class, Status, and Party Influences on Occupational Closure, 1902-1919." *Sociological Quarterly* 51, no. 4 (2010): 550-75.

Weller, Charles D. "Antitrust Joint Ventures and the End of the AMA's Contract Practice Ethics: New Ways of Thinking about the Health Care Industry." *North Carolina Central Law Journal* 14, no. 1 (1983): 3-32.

Weller, Charles D. "'Free Choice' as a Restraint of Trade in American Health Care Delivery and Insurance." *Iowa Law Review* 69, no. 5 (1984): 1351-92.

Wells, Wyatt. *Antitrust and the Formation of the Postwar World*. New York: Columbia University Press, 2002.

White, Richard. *The Republic for Which It Stands. The United States during Reconstruction and the Gilded Age, 1865-1896*. New York: Oxford University Press, 2017.

"Who Names the Ford Hospital Wins Big Honors." *Pittsburgh Press*, July 5, 1914.

Wiegand, Wayne. "Dewey Declassified: A Revelatory Look at the 'Irrepressible Reformer.'" *American Libraries* 27, no. 1 (1996): 54-60.

"Wild Youth Warned to Check Fast Pace." *Pittsburgh Press*, January 26, 1932.

Williams, J. Whitridge. "A Criticism of Certain Tendencies in American Obstetrics." *New York State Journal of Medicine* 22 (1922): 493–99.

Williams, J. Whitridge. "Medical Education and the Midwife Problem in the United States." *Journal of the American Medical Association* 58, no. 1 (1912): 1–7.

Williams, Simon, and Michael Calnan. "The 'Limits' of Medicalization? Modern Medicine and the Lay Populace in 'Late' Modernity." *Social Science and Medicine* 46, no. 12 (1996): 1609–20.

Woolley, Edward Mott. "A Successful Surgeon's Own Story." *American Magazine* 81, no. 6 (1916): 22–24, 80–82.

"Work of Drs. Mayo Now Perpetuated for People's Good." *St. Louis Star and Times*, September 19, 1917.

Wright, Chris. "Taylorism Reconsidered: The Impact of Scientific Management within the Australian Workplace." *Labour History* 64 (1993): 34–53.

Wright, Henry. "Dimensions of Private Rooms." *Modern Hospital* 19, no. 4 (1922): 278–80.

Wright-Mendoza, Jessie. "The 1910 Report That Disadvantaged Minority Doctors." *JSTOR Daily*, May 3, 2019. https://daily.jstor.org/the-1910-report-that-unintentionally-disadvantaged-minority-doctors/.

Young, H. B. "On the Economics of New Medical Titles." *American Medicine* 19 (1913): 660–61.

Index

allopathy, 99, 104, 106, 143, 154, 162. *See also* medical sects
American Civil War, 110
American College of Surgeons (ACS), 8, 12, 92, 108, 139-42, 167; community health meetings organized by, 115-38, 153; hospital standardization program of, 13-14, 51, 67, 74-85, 88, 117; marketing efforts of, 14, 115-26; minimum standard set by, 84, 88; surgical standardization by, 74-82, 154
American Hospital Association (AHA), 8, 61, 88, 140
American Medical Association (AMA), 8, 14-15, 43, 67, 106, 118, 133, 137; Bureau of Medical Economics of, 147; Council on Medical Education of, 95; Flexner Report and, 92-93, 95, 108; monopoly prosecution of, 14, 139-62; race and, 87-88, 112
American Medicine Mobilizes (Rorty), 156
American Railway Association, 122-23
anti-vaccination, 128
Arnold, Thurman, 142-43, 151-53
assembly line: childbirth and, 26-31; digestion and, 21-24; medicine and, 12-13, 49-50, 52-53

Babson, Roger, 47
Bacon, Asa, 63-64
Bancroft, Frederick, 1-4, 71
Battle Creek Sanitarium, 21-22
Behrens, P. W., 64
Bernheim, Bertram, 157

Besley, Frederic, 126-27
Bevan, Arthur Dean, 95
Black Hospital Movement, 88-89
Blalock, Alfred, 59
body: efficiency and, 45; processing and, 20-30
Bonner, Thomas, 108
Borden Milk Company, 146
Boss Tweed, 102
Bowman, John, 118-20, 126-27, 129
Brady, James, 124
Brandeis, Louis, 9, 73, 102, 152; "bigness" and, 94, 152; scientific management and, 7-9. *See also* monopoly
Braverman, Harry, 8
Brown, Richard, E., 166
Bryan, William Jennings, 104
Bulletin of the American College of Surgeons, 74, 78
Bynum, William Dallas, 104

Cabot, Hugh, 53, 154, 160
Cabot, Richard, 33-34, 53, 55
California League for the Conservation of Public Health, 84
California Medical College in Los Angeles, 96
California State Journal of Medicine, 78
cancer: Henry Ford and, 44-46; marketing and, 125, 130-31, 133
capitalism, 7-8, 12-13; efficiency and, 14, 158; industrial, 14, 40, 42, 46, 49; medical, 92-95, 107-9, 142-62; monopoly, 12; racial, 46-47, 60-61; socialized, 146; welfare, 48

Carnegie, Andrew, 7, 40, 45, 73
Carnegie Bulletin Number 4, Medical Education in the United States and Canada: A Report to the Carnegie Foundation for the Advancement of Teaching. See Flexner Report
Carnegie Foundation for the Advancement of Teaching, 61–62, 82, 101, 120, 166; Flexner Report commissioned by, 13, 72, 92–93, 95, 108–9, 111–12
cartelization, 151–52
Catholic Hospital Association, 83, 117
Cattaraugus County Medical Society, 145
Century of Progress Exposition, 125
Chapin, Christy Ford, 15
Chaplin, Charlie, 85
Chicago Maternity Center, 28–29
childbirth, 12–13, 24–29
class: childbirth and, 27–29; efficiency and, 2, 5–6, 7–8, 11, 68, 70; Flexner on, 72–73, 93, 100, 105–9; group practice and, 149; Henry Ford Hospital and, 40, 48, 55–58, 61; silent majority and, 11, 127, 134, 167, 191n44
Clinical Congress of North America, 75, 78–79
closed staff, 51–54, 144–45
Cochrane, Archie, 7, 163–64, 167
Codman, Ernest Amory, 4, 17–19, 70, 79, 81, 164, 167; Bone Cancer Registry of, 69
color line, 59–60, 109–13
Colwell, N. P., 95
Committee on the Costs of Medical Care (CCMC), 136, 153–55, 160
community health meetings, 115–17; American College of Surgeons' strategies for, 117–26; audience composition of, 127–28; cancer at, 130; messaging and, 126–27; personal health and, 129–33; surgical prowess and, 134–35
Coolidge, Calvin, 167
Craig, Allan, 116, 127
Crowell, Bowman, 134
Crowther, Samuel, 54

Davis, Michael M., 32, 146, 148
death panels, 166
de Kruif, Paul, 28
DeLee, Joseph B, 26–27, 29; celebrity status of, 27; filmmaking practices of, 29–31. *See also* prophylactic forceps operation

democracy: American College of Surgeons and, 77–80, 133–34; American Medical Association and, 144; efficiency and, 6, 10–13, 29, 73–74, 158, 167–68; Flexner on, 93, 94, 100–101, 104, 106, 108; race and, 86–90, 113, 132–33
Detroit Academy of Surgery, 55
Detroit General Hospital, 43
Detroit Medical Society, 52
Dewey, Melville, 9, 171n29
Dickinson, Robert Latou, 4
Dick-Read, Grantly, 16, 25, 28–29
digestion, 12–13, 21–24, 45
District Medical Society, 149
Doctor, The (Fildes), 160
doctor-patient relationship, 143–44, 158–62, 168
Du Bois, W. E. B., 60, 109–11, 113, 127
Duden, Barbara, 24–25
Dunott, Daniel, 122

East Baton Rouge Medical Society, 145
education, 3, 5, 13, 91, 93–94; democracy and, 100–101, 104; medical, 3, 13, 97–113
Effectiveness and Efficiency (Cochrane), 163
efficiency, 1, 3, 7–10, 22; democracy and, 6, 10–13, 29, 73–74, 158, 167–68; doctor-patient relationship and, 143–44, 158–62; hospital, 3–4, 31–37, 49–60, 63–90; science and, 5, 98–99; socialism and, 143–44, 146; surgical, 3, 71
El Centro Asturiano, 148
El Centro Español, 148
eugenics: childbirth and, 27–29; Henry Ford and, 46
evidence-based medicine, 163–64

factories: effectiveness and, 33–37, 98–100; efficiency and, 6, 46, 50, 56–57; medical models of, 32–33, 35–37, 66
fascism, 146
fees: flat, 54–58, 145; fee-for-service model of, 54–55, 143–45, 150
Fight for Life, 28
Fildes, Luke, 160
Finney, J. M. T., 75
Fishbein, Morris, 139, 147, 151, 153, 158–59
Fletcher, Horace, 22, 45

Flexner, Abraham, 4, 69, 89, 120, 167; democracy and, 73, 100–101, 105–9; educational reform and, 5, 72, 91–94; race and, 87, 89, 109–13. *See also* Flexner Report
Flexner, Simon, 92, 106–7
Flexner Report, 12–14, 75, 77, 86, 87, 89, 95–100, 120, 186n9; Black medical schools and, 109–13; history of medical education and, 97–98; legacy of, 93, 95, 108; "poor boy" and, 14, 105–8, 113; proprietary schools and, 96–98
Forbes, Edgar Allan, 120
Ford, Henry, 5, 7, 40, 117, 151; anti-Semitism and, 40, 94; eugenic and racial beliefs of, 46–47; medical beliefs of, 1, 24, 45; philanthropy of, 44–46, 57–59; populism and, 41, 46, 56; rationalization and, 19–20
Fordism, 8, 11, 40–41, 47, 94, 108, 143, 166
Ford Model T, 19, 39, 41, 50, 61, 117; pricing of, 56–57
Ford Motor Company, 5, 19–20, 39, 61; $5 day-wage and, 43, 46–48, 61; Great Depression and, 151–52; "industrial sanitorium" and, 47; Sociological Department of, 46–48, 57
Foster, William Trufant, 150, 155
Freedman's Bureau, 111
free enterprise, 146–47
Freidson, Eliot, 166

Garceau, Oliver, 145, 156–57
Gates, Bill, 15
Georgia College of Eclectic Medicine and Surgery, 96
Germ theory, 1, 24, 116–17, 174n23
Gilbreth, Frank, 1–6, 8–10, 18–19, 51; standardization and, 51, 66–67, 70–72, 76, 84
Gilbreth, Lillian, 1–6, 8–10, 19
GlaxoSmithKlein, 168
Goldwater, Sigismund S., 4, 147
Gramsci, Antonio, 40
Great Depression, 9, 14; American College of Surgeons and, 133–37; American Medical Association and, 157–58; efficiency and, 143–46; Ford and, 59–61; hospitals and, 90; overproduction and, 102–3, 150–52
Green, H. M., 86, 87, 88, 89
Gresham's Law, 104

Group Health Association (GHA), 142, 149
group practice, 33–34, 52–54. *See also* lodge practice

Haber, Samuel, 9
happiness minutes, 18–19, 173n7
Harris County Medical Society, 149
Henry Ford Hospital, 13, 40–46, 48–62, 145, 150; design of, 49–50; Ford's influence on, 51, 54–58; race at, 59–61
"Home-made Hospital Appliances" column, 64–65, 71, 73, 80
Hornsby, John, 4, 33, 35
hospitals: design of, 35–37, 49–50; efficiency at, 3–4, 31–37, 49–60, 63–80; standardization of, 74–85, 81–90, 117
Houdini, Harry, 116
Howard University, 109, 111–13
Howell, Thomas, 4
How the Fires of the Body Are Fed (ACS film), 128, 131
Hubbard, George, 111

Illich, Ivan, 7, 165
Itinerary of a Breakfast, The (Kellogg), 23–24

Jackson, Algernon Brashear, 87
Jewson, Nicholas, 166
Jim Crow, 110
Johns Hopkins: hospital, 42, 51, 53, 83; medical school, 29, 92–93, 98, 102, 107
Jolly, Robert, 136
Jones, Philip Mills, 78–80, 121
Journal of the American Medical Association, 104, 156–57
Journal of the National Medical Association, 87, 89

Kahn, Albert, 41, 49
Kellogg, John Harvey, 21–24, 45
Kellogg, Will Keith, 21
Kenney, John, 89
Kingsbury, John, 146

Lee, John, 46
Liebold, Ernest, 49
lodge practice, 147–48, 154
Longworth, Alice Roosevelt, 27–28
Lorentz, Pare, 28

INDEX   223

MacEachern, Malcolm, 124–25
Magill, Thomas, 165
marketing, 115–25, 156–57
Martin, Edward, 81
Martin, Franklin: American College of Surgeons and, 74, 78–83; community health meetings and, 123, 125–27, 130; health care costs and, 136–37
Massachusetts General Hospital, 17–18, 33, 43, 53, 70
maternal mortality, 25–26
Mayo, Charles, 4, 33–34, 42, 53, 133
Mayo, William James, 4, 33, 42, 53
Mayo Clinic, 13, 20, 42, 53; architecture of, 35–37; fees at, 54–55; group practice at, 32–34, 52, 144
McClure, Roy, 52, 59
McKeown, Thomas, 7, 165
Means, James, 161
medical sects, 3, 66, 67, 77, 97, 99, 105, 155. *See also* allopathy
Meharry Medical College, 109, 111–13
Metcalf, William, 43–44
Milbank, Albert, 146
Milbank Fund, 145
milk bottle wars, 145–46
Modern Hospital (journal), 4, 32, 62, 101. *See also* "Home-made Hospital Appliances" column
Modern School, A (Flexner), 91
Modern Times (film), 85
monopoly: AMA as, 15, 142–57; efficiency and, 6, 8, 10–11, 143, 158–62
Moulinier, Charles, 83, 117, 120, 122, 131
Mr. Flexner's School, 91
muckraking, 6, 102–3, 156
Murphy, John, 74, 78
Murray, "Alfalfa" Bill, 145

National Association for the Advancement of Colored People (NAACP), 90
National Civic Organization, 46
National Health Conference, 154
National Hospital Association, 88–90
National Industrial Recovery Act (NIRA), 150–52
nationalized healthcare, 143, 149, 155
National Medical Association (NMA), 12, 86, 88–90

National Physicians' Committee, 160
"Negro Hospital Renaissance, The" (Kenney), 89
Neupert, Carl von, 133
New Deal, 28, 149, 155, 158
new social history of medicine, 7–10, 18; anti-institutionalist bent of, 163–68; Flexner and, 92–93, 108
New York Giants, 9–10
New York Hospital, 1–2, 4, 71

Oklahoma Farmer's Union, 145
One Scar or Many (ACS film), 128
organized medicine, 8, 106; American Medical Association as, 152–53, 160; critiques of, 155–57, 166; Group Health Association and, 149; Tampa Municipal Hospital and, 140–45
Our Master's Voice (Rorty), 156
overproduction, 102–4; doctor quality related to, 103–4; underproduction versus, 109. *See also* Great Depression

Palin, Sarah, 166
personalized medicine, 168
Philadelphia County Medical Society, 17–18
Philadelphia Phillies, 9–10
philanthropy, 40–41, 44–46, 57–59; Black medical schools and, 111–12; charity and, 59–60, 91, 112–13; color line and, 59–60, 109–13; Henry Ford on, 45–46
Plummer, Henry S., 35
Polo Grounds, 9–10
Pool, Eugene, 1–4, 71
populism, 42, 46
precision medicine, 168
Principles of Scientific Management (Taylor), 71
Pritchett, Henry: Carnegie Foundation and, 101, 120; Flexner Report and, 92, 95, 102, 106–7, 111, 113
processing, 4, 17–20; childbirth as, 24–31; digestion as, 21–24; "happiness minutes" and, 18–19; hospitals and, 17; Mayo Clinic and, 31–37; product of, 12; standardization and, 18
professionalization: medical, 6–8, 13, 18, 92–93, 166–67
Prohibition, 127, 167
prophylactic forceps operation, 26–27, 29
Purinton, Edward, 9, 171n32

racism, 11–12; Henry Ford Hospital and, 59–61; hospital standardization and, 86–90; lodge practice and, 147–48; medical education and, 109–13
Reconstruction, 89
reproduction: industrial revolution and, 24–25; film and, 30–31
Reverby, Susan, 166
Reward of Courage (Cancer Society film), 130
Rockefeller, John D., 7, 40
Rockefeller Foundation, 61, 93, 109, 111–12, 166
Rockefeller Institute for Medical Research, 107
Roman, C. V., 89
Roosevelt, Franklin, 28, 149, 155
Rorty, James, 156–57
Rosenberg, Charles, 21, 166
Rosenwald, Julius, 113
Roses, Allen, 168
Rosner, David, 166
Royal College of Surgeons, 81

Sanders, Lisa, 168
Savitt, Todd, 111, 112
scientific management, 7–9, 173n18
Shadid, Michael, 145
Sherman Antitrust Act, 68, 142, 152
Shortcliffe, Edward, 167
Shoudy, Loyal, 132
Shryock, Richard, 155
Sigerist, Henry, 155, 162
silent majority, 11, 127, 134, 167, 191n44
Slobe, Frederick, 84
social clubs: health care and, 147–48
social gospel, 46, 61
socialism, 144–47, 158
sovietism, 147, 159
sports: efficiency and, 9–10
Squier, J. Bentley, 133, 136
standardization, 12–13, 68–73, 104; American College of Surgeons Hospital program of, 74–85, 88, 117; Black hospitals and, 86–90; critiques of, 78–80, 84–85; democracy and, 73–74, 77–79, 104, 144, 158–62; education and, 72, 93–94, 100–101; hospital, 81–90; invention and, 65–67, 72–73, 143; marketing of, 115–26; science and, 69, 99–101; surgical, 74–82, 154

Standard Oil, 5, 6, 68, 73–74, 106
Starr, Paul, 7, 18, 166
Steffans, Lincoln, 102
Stomach, The (Kellogg), 21–22
Surgery, Gynecology and Obstetrics. See *Bulletin of the American College of Surgeons*
Surgical Clinics of John B. Murphy, MD, at Mercy Hospital, Chicago (annual publication), 79
Sweet, Ossian, 60

Tammany Hall, 102
Tampa Municipal Hospital: kerfuffle at, 139–42; and lodge practice, 147–49
Tarbell, Ida, 6, 68
Taylor, Frederick Winslow, 3, 5, 7, 40, 71, 84
Taylorism, 8, 40, 143, 166
Taylor Society, 3
Thirkield, Wilbur, 111–12
Thomas, Vivien, 59
Tomes, Nancy, 15
Trinity Hospital, 145
twilight sleep, 9
Tylenol, 168

United States of America, Appellants, v. The American Medical Association, A Corporation; The Harris County Medical Society, An Association, et al., Appellees, 142–43, 149–53
University of Louisville Medical Department, 106
US Steel, 5, 73, 94

Veblen, Thorsten, 156

Washington, Booker T., 89, 110
Wayne County Medical Society, 55
Welch, William, 107
welfare, 46, 59
wet clinics, 78–79
Wharton, Edith, 9
Williams, J. Whitridge, 29
World's Work (journal), 96, 120

Ybor City, 147–48
Young, H. B., 74, 77

www.ingramcontent.com/pod-product-compliance
Lightning Source LLC
Chambersburg PA
CBHW020236170426
43202CB00008B/105